Foundations of Plant Pathology

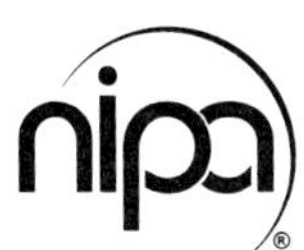

NIPA® GENX ELECTRONIC RESOURCES & SOLUTIONS P. LTD.
New Delhi-110 034

About the Author

Dr. Sanjeev Kumar is an Assistant Professor in the Department of Plant Pathology, Office of Dean,Faculty of Agriculture, Jawaharlal Nehru Krishi Vishwavidyalaya, Jabalpur, Madhya Pradesh. He is a very sincere and enthusiastic teacher. He has taught with dedication to the satisfaction of students in many undergraduate, graduate and doctoral programs and has been actively involved in all educational activities. Dr. Kumar has mentored 23 MSc students and 2 of his PhD students and is also actively involved in their research and extension activities. As a researcher, he has been involved in his eight major research projects sponsored by ICAR, NATP, TSP and JICA, Japan. He has published 75 research and review articles, 25 book chapters, 105 popular articles, 1 research bulletin, and 3 technical brochures. He is an active member of more than six national and international societies. He is fellow of Indian Phytopathological Society, IARI New Delhi, Indian Society of Mycology and Phytopathology, Udaipur, Rajasthan, Society for Biocontrol Advancement, Banglulu. He has participated in many conferences, symposiums, workshops and presented papers. He also attended the World Soybean Research Conference in Durban, South Africa.

Dr. Kumar has authored twelve books entitled Plant Pathogens and Principles of Plant Pathology, Horticultural Crop Diseases: Identification and Management, Diseases of Field Crop and their Integrated Management, Pesticides and Plant Protection Appliances, Diseases of Field and Horticultural Crop and Their Management-II, Fundamentals of Plant Pathology, Integrated Management; Principles & Practices,Chemicals & Botanicals in Plant Diease Managment published by New India. Publishing Agency, Pithampura, New Delhi and Textbook of Field and Horticultural Crop Diseases and Their Management-I published by, Brillion Publishing, Desh Bandhu Gupta Road, Karol Bagh, New Delhi-110005, and his three practical manuals. His research interests include pulse pathology and biological control.

Foundations of Plant Pathology

Sanjeev Kumar
Assistant Professor/Scientist
Department of Plant Pathology
Officc of Dean, Faculty of Agriculture
Jawaharlal Nehru Krishi Vishwa Vidyalaya
Jabalpur-482004, Madhya Pradesh, India

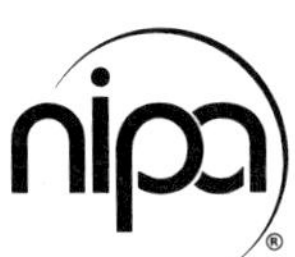

NIPA® GENX ELECTRONIC RESOURCES & SOLUTIONS P. LTD.
New Delhi-110 034

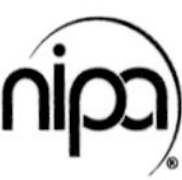

NIPA® GENX ELECTRONIC RESOURCES & SOLUTIONS P. LTD.

101,103, Vikas Surya Plaza, CU Block
L.S.C. Market, Pitam Pura, New Delhi-110 034
Ph : +91-11-43860225, Mob.: +91 9717133558, 9540816132
E-mail: newindiapublishingagency@gmail.com
Website: www.nipaersources.com

Print ISBN: 978-93-58874-89-1

ebook ISBN: 978-93-58878-90-5

Composed and Designed by NIPA®.

Preface

It has been observed that compliance with the various provisions of the National Education Policy 2020 requires a paradigm shift in academic regulation. ICAR continues to work on the reforms needed to ensure the quality of agricultural education. The council appointed 'Sixth Deans Committee' to review and restructure the graduate curriculum. The Under Graduate Agricultural Education Programs has been reorganized and new courses have been introduced. The curriculum has been restructured to enable students to acquire knowledge, approach entrepreneurship and improve their employability and skills to prepare for international competitiveness. This 'Foundations of Plant Pathology' book has been carefully written for the Undergraduate class and is fully compliant with the latest syllabus. The purpose of producing this text is to provide basic and fresh facts to enable students to introduce the scientific foundations and basics of plant pathology in this course. Great care was taken to present facts appropriate to the student's level and grade the content accordingly. The text of the book is clear, well presented and arranged according to the curriculum. Infohive aims to inspire young minds to learn new things and expand their skills.Chapters are designed to lead to comprehensive learning, with key concepts to help develop students' investigative skills. Each chapter ends with a sample question paper. Sample papers contain all of the syllabus's important topics and frequently answered questions, making them thorough revision aids. Frequent use of them strengthens knowledge, sharpens reasoning abilities, and dispels uncertainty, resulting in a more sophisticated comprehension of the material.

I make no claims of originality in the creation of this book and have had the help of numerous books, magazines, bulletins, and electronic resources. We would like to express our sincere gratitude to the pioneers past and present in the field of plant pathology.

The book entitled Foundations of Plant Pathology written by me is dedicated to my parents, who sacrificed everything to give me the most and best education possible, to my wife, 'Archana' whose love and support have been the most precious things to me throughout our life together, andm who helped me in many facets of preparation of this and of previous books and finally, to “Saumya” and “Adyan”, our youngest children, who, someday, when they read their names in the book, may be reassured of “Papa” love for them, and may feel proud of their father. In this endeavor, omissions and errors will inevitably be found, and I accept responsibility for factual errors. Teachers and students are invited to comment on the book and make suggestions for further improvement.

January, 2025 **Sanjeev Kumar**
Jabalpur

Contents

Fun Time

Acervulus: A saucer-shaped, spore-producing body of a fungus embedded in host tissue.

Actinomycetes Filamentous bacteria that produce several antibiotics and give soil its earthy smell.

Active ingredient: In pesticides, the chemical responsible for the desired effect.

Aggressiveness: Virulent forms of pathogen cause differing degrees of symptom severity.

Alternate Host One of two kinds of plants on which a parasitic fungus must develop to complete its life cycle.

Anamorph: Asexual stage of a fungus.

Antagonism: The counteraction between organisms or groups of organisms.

Antibiotic: A complex chemical substance produced by one microorganism that inhibits or kills other microorganisms.

Antiseptic: A substance that prevents, retards, or destroys microorganisms.

Apothecium: An open, cuplike, or saucer-shaped sexual fungal fruiting body containing asci.

Asexual: Vegetative without sex organs, sex cells, or sexual spores, as the anamorph of a fungus.

Autoecious: The need of only one host for completing the life cycle of a rust.

Avirulence: The inability of a pathogen to cause disease.

Bactericide: A compound toxic to bacteria.

Biotroph: A plant pathogenic fungus that requires living host cells i.e. an obligate parasite.

Blotch: A blot or spot, usually superficial and irregular in shape and size, on leaves, shoots and fruit.

Callus: Parenchyma tissue that grows over a wound or graft and protects it against drying or other injury.

Chemotherapy: Treatment of disease by chemicals (chemothera-peutants) working internally. Chemical agent has toxic effect directly or indirectly on the pathogens without injury to the host plant.

Chlamydospore: A thick-walled asexual resting spore formed by the modification of a fungus hypha.

Cleistothecium: Closed, usually spherical, ascus-containing structure of powdery mildew fungi. A sexual fruiting structure.

Conidiophore: The specialized fungal hyphal branch that bears the conidium.

Collateral host: The wild host of same families of a pathogen is called as collateral host.

Curative Chemical control method aimed at inhibiting the development of an established infection.

Diagnostic: Distinctive. A distinguishing characteristic serving to identify or determine the presence of a disease or other condition.

Disease: Any deviation in the general health, or physiology or function of plant or plant parts, is recognized as a disease.

Disease cycle: The chain of events involved in disease development.

Disinfectant: Any agent for destroying the causal agent of disease after infection.

Disinfestant: Any agent that removes, kills, or inactivates diseasc-causing organisms *before* they can cause infection.

Enphytotic: Plant disease that causes about the same amount of injury each year.

Environment: The external conditions and influences that surround living organisms.

Epidemiology: The study of factors influencing the initiation, development, and spread of infectious disease.

Eradication: Control of disease by eliminating the pathogen after it is already established.

Escape: Plants in a given population that remain free of disease where it is prevalent, although they possess no natural inherent resistance to the disease.

Etiolation: Yellowing and long, spindly growth as a result of insufficient light.

Etiology: The description of the cause of disease.

Exclusion: Control of disease by preventing its introduction (e.g., by quarantines) into disease-free areas.

Facultative Parasite: An organism that is ordinarily saprophytic but under proper conditions may be parasitic.

Facultative Saprophyte: An organism that is ordinarily parasitic but under proper conditions may be saprophytic.

Fruiting Body: Any of various complex, spore-bearing fungal structures.

Fumigant: Vapor-active chemical used in the gaseous phase to kill or inhibit the growth of microorganisms or other pests.

Fungi Imperfecti: A major group of fungi for which no sexual production of spores is known.

Fungicide: An agent that inhibits or kills fungi.

Fungistat: A chemical or physical agent that prevents fungi from developing but does not kill them.

Haploid: The chromosome number of the gametophytic genera-tion or phase or having a single complete set of chromosomes.

Haustorium: A modified mycelial branch that grows into a plant cell, makes intimate contact with the protoplast, and absorbs food.

Hemibiotroph: A plant pathogenic fungus that initially requires living host cells but after killing the host cell grows on the dead and dying cells.

Heteroecious: Requiring two or more unrelated hosts for completing the life cycle of a rust.

Heterothallic: Producing fusing gametes on separate and distinct mycelia.

Hemiparasites: Parasitic plants that have chlorophyl and can make some of their own sugar but still rely on thier host for water and other nutrients.

Holoparasites: Parasitic plants that do not have chlorphyl and rely on thier host for all nutrients.

Homothalic: Producing fusing gametes on the same mycelium.

Host: The plant on or in which a parasite lives and from which it obtains its food.

Hyaline Clear, translucent.

Hypersensitive: Plant responds to pathogen infection by quickly killing the infected cells, blocking the advance of the pathogen.

Hyperplasia: A symptom due to an abnormal increase in the number of individual cells.

Hypertrophy: An symptom due to an abnormal increase in the size of individual cells.

Hyphae: Fungal filaments which collectively form the mycelium of a fungus.

Hypoplasia: The underdevelopment of cells, tissues, or organs.

Immune: Cannot be infected by a given pathogen.

Immunity: A relationship between a plant and a causal agent in which the plant does not become diseased.

Incubation period: The period of time between penetration of a pathogen to the host and the first appearance of symptoms on the plant.

Indexing: Determining presence of disease in a plant by removing buds or other parts for inoculation of a susceptible indicator plant that exhibits specific symptoms of a transmissible disease.

Infection: The initiation and establishment of a parasite within a host plant.

Infection court: Specific area on a plant where a pathogen gains entrance to the host.
Inoculum: That portion of pathogen which is transferred to plant and cause disease.
Inoculation: The process of transferring inoculum to host.
Inoculum density: The number of infective units in a given volume or area.
Inoculum potential: The growth or threshold of fungus available for colonization at host.
Invasion: The penetration and spread of a pathogen in the host.
Intercellular: Between the cells.
Intracellular: Within the cells.
Latent: Present but not manifest or visible, as a symptomless infection.
Lesion: A local injury or delimited diseased area.
Macrocyclic: Rusts that produce all five spore types.
Microcyclic: Rusts that lack one or more of the five spore types.
Mechanical transmission: Virus transmission from plant to plant by infected plant sap.
Monocycic disease: A disease where only one disease cycle is completed each year or growing season.
Multiple cycle disease: Some pathogens specially a fungus, can complete a number of life cycles within one crop season of the host plant and the disease caused by such pathogens is called multiple cycle disease e.g. wheat rust, rice blast, late blight of potato etc.
Mycelium: The mass of interwoven threads (hyphae) making up the vegetative body of a fungus.
Mycoplasma: Degenerate bacteria that do not have cell walls. Mycoplasmas are smaller than bacteria but larger than viruses. They cause animal and human diseases.
Necrosis: A symptom marked by rapid death of the host or parts of the host.
Necrotroph: A pathogenic fungus that kills the host and survives on the dying and dead cells.
Nematicide: chemical or physical agent that kills, inhibits, or protects against nematodes.
Obligate: Necessary; obliged.
Obligate parasite: An obligate parasite is an organism that can live only on living tissue.
Parasite: An organism that lives within or upon another living organism from which it derives nourishment and in which it may cause various degrees of injury.
Parasitism: The phenomenon of the growth of one organism, the parasite, at the expense of another, the host.
Pathogen: An entity, usually a micro-organism that can cause the disease.
Pathogenicity: An entity's capacity for producing a disease.
Pathogenesis: It is a process caused by an infectious agent (pathogen) when it comes in contact with a susceptible host.
Pathology: The study of disease.
Perithecium: A round to flask-shaped, thick-walled spore case containing asci and with an ostiole (pore).
Pesticide: Any chemical or physical agent that destroys pests (e.g., fungicide, insecticide, miticide).
Phytoplasma: Microorganisms found in phloem tissue that resemble mycoplasmas in all respects except that they cannot yet be grown on artificial nutrient media. Formerly known as mycoplasmalike organism (MLO).
Plasmodium: A naked, multinucleate, vegetative (fungal) body capable of amoeboid motion.
Preventative: Chemical control method aimed at preventing infection of the pathogen.
Primary infection: The first infection of a plant by the over wintering or over summering of the pathogen.
Primary Inoculum: Inoculum, usually from an overwintering source, that initiates disease in the field, as opposed to inoculum that spreads disease during the season.

Propagule: The part of an organism that may be spread so as to reproduce the organism.

Prophylaxis: Methods used to preserve health and prevent spread of disease.

Protectant: A chemical applied to a plant surface in advance of the pathogen to prevent infection.

Pustule: A local elevation of the epidermis that may rupture to expose the causal agent (e.g., rust, smut, white rust, etc.).

Pycnidium: The asexual, globose or flask-shaped fruiting body of fungi-producing conidia.

Quarantine: Regulation forbidding sale or shipment of plants or plant parts, usually to prevent disease, insect, nematode, or weed invasion of an area.

Resistance: The sum of the qualities of the host and causal agent that retard the activities of the causal agent.

Rust: Used to describe a particular fungus, any of its stages or the disease caused by any of the stages.

Sanitation: Destroying all infested and infected plant parts during the season.

Saprophyte: An organism that derives its nourishment from dead organic matter.

Secondary Infection: Infection resulting from the spread of infectious material produced after a primary infection.

Sign : The structure of the pathogen itself.

Single cycle disease: This type of disease is referred to those caused by the pathogen (fungi) that can complete only one life cycle in one crop season of the host plant. e.g. downy mildew of rapeseed, club root of crucifers, sclerotinia blight of brinjal etc.

Spiroplasma: A single-celled, wall-less, spiral, filamentous organism associated with corn stunt and citrus stubborn disease.

Sporangiophore: A sporangium-bearing hypha.

Spore: A fungal reproductive unit or seed that serves as an agent of dispersal and propagation.

Susceptibility The sum of the qualities of a plant and causal agent that allows the development of the causal agent.

Symbiosis: A mutually beneficial association of two or more different kinds of organisms.

Symptoms: The external and internal reaction or alterations of a plant as a result of disease.

Systemic: Pertaining to a disease in which an infection leads to general spread throughout the plant body. Also, a chemical that spreads internally through a plant.

Systemic aquired resistance: Whole plant resistance response that occurs following an earlier localized exposure to a pathogen.

Teliomorph: Sexual stage of a fungus.

Teliospore: Thick-walled resting spore produced by some fungi, notably rusts and smuts, that germinates to form a basidium.

Thallus: The vegetative body of the lower plant that has not differentiated into stems and leaves.

Tolerance: Ability of the plant to endure the development of the parasite without showing marked symptoms of disease.

Transgenic plants: Plants that have been genetically manipulated to express a gene from a different species.

Tumor: A swelling or protuberance.

Vector: An agent, such as an insect, nematode, or fungus, that may transmit a pathogen.

Viroid: An infectious nucleic acid without a protein coat that causes potato spindle tuber or chrysanthemum stunt.

Virulence: The degree of infectivity of a given pathogen.

Viruliferous: Capable of transmitting a virus.

Water-soaked: Describing plants or lesions that appear wet and dark and are usually sunken and translucent.

1

Introduction to Plant Pathology

Plant Pathology

The term Plant Pathology is derived from greek words- *pathos* (suffering) + *logos* (study) i.e. the study of the suffering plant. Plant Pathology has two phases broadly-

- **Science**- Understanding of the disease i.e. the theoretical consideration of the suffering plants and how do pathogens invade, how do plants defend themselves, what causes symptoms etc.
- **Art**- The application of the science to the field problems i.e. Diagnosis and Control.

Plant pathology or phytopathology is the branch of agricultural, botanical or biological science which deals with the cause, etiology, resulting in losses and management methods of plant diseases.

Plant pathology can also be defined as the study of the nature, cause and prevention of plant diseases. Plant pathology is related to most of the old and new sciences like biology, physics, chemistry, physiology, mathematics, genetics, soil science, biochemistry, biotechnology etc.

Study of plant pathology includes the study of sciences *viz*, microbiology, bacteriology, virology, mycology, nematology, protozology, phycology, unfavorable , environmental factors, nutritional deficiencies and flowering plant parasites.

1. Microbiology: Study of microorganisms
2. Bacteriology: Study of bacteria
3. Virology: Study of viruses
4. Mycology: Study of fungi
5. Nematology: Study of nematode
6. Protozology: Study of protozoa
7. Phycology: Study of algae.

Major Objectives

1. To study biotic (living), mesobiotic and abiotic (non-living and environmental) causes of diseases or disorders.
2. To study the mechanisms of disease development by pathogens.
3. To study the plant (host)-pathogen interaction in relation to environment.
4. To develop methods of management of plant diseases.

Scope of Plant Pathology

- Field surveys to determine disease prevalence and incidence.
- Recordings of newly emerging diseases of economic importance, including details and extent of outbreaks.
- Assessment of losses due to various economically important diseases.
- Studies of the etiology, symptoms, predisposition, and recurrence of such diseases.
- Identification of suitable and economical methods to manage economically important crop diseases.
- Support for breeding disease-resistant varieties.
- Training of advisors and subject matter experts to bridge the gap between pathologists and farmers for better crop production.

Importance of Plant Pathology in Agriculture

- Plant pathology has advanced the knowledge to protect the crop from losses due to diseases.
- Most of the diseases with known disease cycle can now be avoided by the modification of cultural practices.
- With the knowledge of mode of disease spread, many diseases of economic importance can now be managed .
- Crop improvement and varietal resistance have been achieved against many diseases through the joint effort of breeder and plant pathologist.
- The science of plant pathology has contributed disease free certified seed production.
- Plant pathology has made it possible to limit the spread of plant diseases from one place to another and from one country to another through appropriate measures and quarantine laws.
- Knowledge of plant pathology allows various preventive measures to be taken to successfully manage disease. These measures are seed treatments, soil treatments and crop rotation.

- Diseases in cold storage can be avoided by taking phytopathological measures, following various disease recommendations to protect stored fruits and vegetables.
- Plant pathology has enabled toxicants to be recognized, removed and utilized through toxicant production, competition and parasitism. Organisms that exert such lethal or harmful effects on other organisms are called antagonists.

Challenges for plant pathology

The challenges for plant pathology are

- To reduce food losses
- To improve food quality
- To safeguarde our environment

Model Practice Questions

A.Objective Questions

a. Multiple Choice Questions

1. The term plant pathology derived from

(a) Greek word (b) American word
(c) French word (d) Latin word

2. The study of the suffering plant is called

(a) Plant Pathology (b) Plant Epidemiology
(c) Plant Taxonomy (d) Plant Physiology

3. Plant pathology is

(a) Science (b) Art
(c) Commerce (d) All

4. The study of the nature, cause and management of plant diseases.

(a) Plant Pathology (b) Plant Breeding
(c) Plant Taxonomy (d) Plant Physiology

5. The study of fungi

(a) Mycology (b) Phycology
(c) Bacteriology (d) Virology

6. The study of algae

(a) Mycology (b) Phycology
(c) Bacteriology (d) Virology

7. The study of the nature, cause and management of plant diseases.
   (a) Plant Pathology (b) Plant Breeding
   (c) Plant Taxonomy (d) Plant Physiology

8. The famous Irish famine of 1845 was caused due to the outbreak of
   (a) Helminthosporiose of rice (b) Stem rust of wheat
   (c) Late blight of potato (d) Downy mildew of grapes

9. In 2005 which pathological scientist got Borlaug award–
   (a) Rattan Lal (b) VL Chopra
   (c) CD Mayee (d) S Nagarajan

10. Renowned scientist Dr. N.E. Borlaug belongs to–
   (a) Agronomy (b) Genetics
   (c) Entomology (d) Plant Pathology

Answer

Q. No.	Answer	Q. No.	Answer
1	(a) Greek word	6	b) Phycology
2	(a) Plant pathology	7	(a) Plant pathology
3	d) All	8	c) Late blight of potato
4	(a) Plant pathology	9	(D) S Nagarajan
5	(a) Mycology	10	(D) Plant pathology

b. True /False

1. Plant pathology has advanced the knowledge to protect the crop from losses due to diseases.
2. Understanding of the plant disease is called science.
3. The science of plant pathology has contributed disease free certified seed production.
4. Crop improvement and varietal resistance have been achieved against many diseases through the joint effort of breeder and plant pathologist.
5. Plant pathology has made it possible to limit the spread of plant diseases from one place to another and from one country to another through appropriate measures and quarantine laws.
6. Most of the diseases with known disease cycle can now be avoided by the modification of cultural practices.
7. Training of advisors and subject matter experts to bridge the gap between pathologists and farmers for better crop production.
8. The application of the science to the field problems i.e. diagnosis and control is called art.

9. Irish famine happen in Ireland due late blight disease of potato.
10. Bengal famine happen in West Bengal due Helminthosporium leaf blight disease of rice.

Q. No.	Answer	Q. No.	Answer
1	True	6	True
2	True	7	True
3	True	8	True
4	True	9	True
5	True	10	True

Subjective Questions

a. Short answer questions

1. What is plant pathology ? Discuss its importance in human welfare.
2. Define plant pathology. Write down the objective and scope of plant pathology in agriculture.
3. Define plant protection. Give its responsibilities to agriculture.
4. Plant pathologists proclaim that plant pathology is a discipline which encompasses both "art" and "science". What do you understand by the "art" of plant pathology?
5. What are the objectives and scope of plant pathology?
6. Write sown the importance of plant pathology in agriculture.

b. Long answer questions

1. What is plant pathology, and what is its scope in modern agriculture?
2. How does plant pathology contribute to global food security?
3. What are the main objectives of plant pathology research and how do they address the challenges of plant diseases?
4. Explain the importance of early disease detection in plant pathology.
5. What is the role of plant pathology in the development of disease-resistant crop varieties?
6. How do environmental factors influence the spread and severity of plant diseases, and what is the role of plant pathology in mitigating these effects?
7. Describe the relationship between plant diseases and the economic impact on agriculture.
8. What are the challenges faced by plant pathologists in the study of emerging plant diseases?

9. What are the key methods used in plant pathology for diagnosing plant diseases?
10. How does integrated pest management (IPM) relate to plant pathology, and why is it important?

2

The Concept of Disease in Plants

Disease

Disease is one of those terms that are very difficult to define. It is realized that disease (literally *dis-ease*) implies *lack of 'comfort'* and therefore, involves *deviation from normal functioning*. From time to time several definitions which have been proposed, in fact descriptive but not simultaneously exclusive. The definitions for the term disease are:

- Disease is a malfunctioning process that is caused by continuous irritation, which results in some suffering producing symptoms.
- Disease is an alteration in one or more of the ordered sequential series of physiological processes culminating in a loss of coordination of energy utilization in a plant as a result of the continuous irritation from the presence or absence of some factor or agent.
- Disease is any morphological or physiological abnormality in a plant or any of its parts caused by continuous irritation and results in economic losses to human beings.
- Any deviation from normal growth or structure of plants that is sufficiently pronounced and permanent to produce visible symptoms or to impair quality and economic value.
- A plant is said to be diseased when there is a harmful deviation from normal functioning of physiological process .

All these definitions indicate that disease;

- Is not a pathogen but it is *caused by a pathogen.*
- It is not symptom but *results in symptoms.*
- It is not a condition as the condition results from disease and is not synonymous with it.
- It is *not an injury.*
- Cannot be infectious, it is actually the pathogen which is infectious.
- Results from continuous irritation.
- And is a malfunctioning process and this result in some suffering and therefore disease is a *pathological process*

Disease *Vs* Injury

- Disease occurs whenever a vital process in the host plant is continuously disrupted.
- Disease is particularly severe when the regulated intake and use of energy is impaired.
- Injury is sometimes confused with disease, and injurious agents are sometimes confused with pathogens. However, this confusion can be avoided.
- Injuries occur when plants are temporarily disturbed. E.g.. By mowers or grasshoppers.
- In contrast, disease occurs when plants are exposed to long-term injury or damage (or, as some authors prefer, "continuous irritation") by pathogens. Examples include wilt fungus and yellow spot fungus.

Concept of Disease in Plants

Old Concept

Plant diseases were viewed as a curse and punishment from god for the wrongs that humans had committed (religious belief and suspertition).Theophrastus, the Greek philosopher, was the first to investigate and record diseases of legumes, cereals, and trees in writing around 300 B.C. His book, "Enquiry into Plants," was written. He talked about his experiences with plant diseases in this book. There was no experimentation behind his experience. His inability to explain his diseases. He believed that diseases were brought about by god's control over the weather. Plant diseases were considered confirmation of God's value. It results from superstitions, occultation, religious beliefs, or bad wind and star moon. For instance, the Romans developed a unique rust god known as Robigo to combat rust diseases in grain crops. They presented sheep and red dogs as sacrifices.This went on for nearly two millennia following Theophrastus. Scientists came to assume that mildews, rust, and other symptoms seen on plants and microorganisms identified on diseased plant were caused by the advent of the compound microscope in the middle of the 1600s, which allowed them to see numerous microorganisms linked with sick plants. Diseases were more often the natural result of plant parts than their cause or effect.

New Concept

Louis Pasteur (1860–63) produced indisputable proof that fermentation is a biological process rather than merely a chemical one and that microbes only develop from pre-existing microorganisms. A plant is considered to be healthy or normal when its physiological processes are carried out to the fullest extent possible by its genetic makeup. When a harmful microbe or unfavorable environmental factor interferes with a plant's or plant part's ability to perform vital functions like respiration, transpiration, photosynthesis, and reproduction, among others, the activities of the cells are disrupted, altered, or inhibited, the cells malfunction or die, and the plant becomes diseased.

The relationship is first invisible and restricted to one or a small number of cells. However, the reaction spreads quickly, and the impacted areas experience changes that are obvious to the unaided eye. These outward manifestations of the disease are its symptom. The quantity of disease in a plant is determined by the visible or other quantifiable negative changes that result from a microbial infection or an adverse environmental condition. Thus, disease in plants is the outcome of a variety of visible and unseen reactions that plant cells and tissues have to a pathogenic microbe or environmental condition. These reactions cause the plant to alter negatively in terms of its form, function, or integrity and may even cause partial impairment or death.

The kind of physiological function that is interrupted first depends on the cells and tissues that are impacted. Root infections, for example, can lead to root rot and impair the plant's ability to absorb water and nutrients from the soil; xylem vessel infections, which occur in all vascular wilts, disrupt water and mineral translocation to the plant's crown; phloem cell infections in leaf veins and stem and shoot bark, which occur in cankers and diseases caused by mollicutes, viruses, and protozoa, disrupt photosynthetic products' downward translocation; Photosynthesis is hampered by foliage infection, such as that caused by blights, leaf spots, mildews, rusts, mosaics, etc. fruit and flower infection interfare reproduction.Even while the majority of infected cells are weakened or die, in certain diseases, such as crown gall, the infection causes the infected cells to divide much more quickly than normal cells (hyperplasia and hypertrophy), which results in abnormal overgrowth (tumors) or malformed organs. Biotic agents, often called pathogens, typically induce disease in plants by secreting compounds such as poisons, enzymes, growth regulators, and other molecules that disrupt the metabolism of plant cells. They also cause disease by taking nutrients from the host cells for their own purposes. Many pathogens can also spread disease by developing and proliferating inside plant vascular bundles, when they obstruct the passage of carbohydrates or water via the corresponding tissues.

Importance of Plant Diseases

1. **Plant diseases may limit the kinds of plants and industries in the area.** Plant diseases can restrict the range of kinds of plants that can be grown over a wide geographic area. For instance, the European grape *Vitis vinifera,* which produces all of the world's premium table and wine

grapes, cannot be cultivated in the Southeast of the United States due to the devastating effects of Pierce's grape diseases. Due to their impact on the quantity and quality of produce available for local processing, plant diseases can also influence the types of agricultural industries and employment levels in a given location. However, the development of new industries that produce equipment, chemicals, and techniques for managing diseased plants is also a result of plant diseases.

2. **Plant diseases reduce the quality and quantity of plant produce.** Plant diseases may cause significant losses by lowering the quality of plant products. For instance, apples with even a 5 percent disease, or apple scab, may reduce the cost in half. In markets where there is only a tiny scarcity of potatoes, the price of potatoes infected with potato scab may not change, but in years where there is even a slight oversupply of product, prices may drop significantly. Plant diseases can result in losses ranging from a small percentage to 100%. Plants and plant products can be affected by diseases that occur in the field, as is the case with the majority of plant diseases, or by diseases that develop during storage, as is the case with the rots of the stored fruits, vegetables, grains, and other plant materials.
3. **Plant diseases may make plants poisonous to humans and animals:** A number of grains, as well as occasionally other seeds and plant products like hay, purees, etc., are often tainted or afflicted with one or more fungus that create mycotoxins, which are extremely dangerous substances. Consuming such goods can cause serious diseases to internal organs, the nervous system, etc. in humans or animals, and even result in death. Certain plant diseases, such as ergot in wheat and rye, contaminate plant products with toxic fruiting structures that render them unfit for human or animal consumption.
4. **Plant diseases may cause financial losses**. Plant diseases can result in financial losses through the following channels. Plants that are resistant to disease may need to be planted by farmers even when these kinds are less productive and profitable for businesses.In order to control a disease, they could need to spray the crop, which would cost money for chemicals, labor, machinery, and storage space.Shippers may incur additional costs if they are required to provide transportation trucks and chilled warehouses. Plant products that are both healthy and diseased might need to be kept apart in order to prevent the disease from spreading, which would increase handling expenses.

The cost of controlling plant diseases is also a direct loss to diseases. Certain plant diseases can be virtually completely controlled using one or more methods, which will result in losses of money equal to the control's cost. But occasionally, like in the case of some small grain diseases, this expense could be just as large as or higher than the crop's anticipated yield.

Plant disease outbreaks with similar far-reaching effects in more recent times are mentioned below

S. No	Major disease outbreaks	Country	Period
1	Late blight of potato (Irish famine)	Ireland	1845–60
2	Powdery and downy mildews	France	1851 and 1878
3	Coffee rust	Ceylon	1870s
4	Fusarium wilts of cotton and flax; Southern bacterial wilt of tobacco	-	Early 1900s
5	Sigatoka leaf spot and Panama disease of banana	Central America	1900–65
6	Leaf spot of rice (Bengal famine)	India	1945
7	Black stem rust of wheat	United State of America	1916, 1935, 1953–54
8	Southern corn leaf blight	United State of America	1970
9	Panama disease of banana	Asia, Australia, and Africa	1990 to present
10	Coffee rust	Central and South America	1960, 2012 to present

Model Practice Questions

A. Objective Questions

1. Deviation from normal functioning of plant is called

(a) Disease (b) Disorder

(c) Pathology (d) Pathogen

2. Disease in plants is caused by

(a) Biotic agents (b) Mesobiotic agents

(c) Abiotic agents (d) All

3. Disorder in plants is caused by

(a) Biotic agents (b) Mesobiotic agents

(c) Abiotic agents (d) All

4. Diseases is

(a) Continnuous irritation (b) Discontinuous irritation

(c) Both (d) None

5. Injury is
   (a) Continnuous irritation (b) Discontinuous irritation
   (c) Both (d) None
6. 'Fungi and Diseases in plants' is written by
   (a) K.C. Mehta (b) B.B. Mundkur
   (c) E.J. Butler (d) R.N. Vasudeva
7. Which among the following are true for disease
   (a) It is not a pathogen but it is *caused by a pathogen.*
   (b) It is not symptom but *results in symptoms.*
   (c) It is *not an injury.*
   (d) All
8. Bengal famine of 1942-43 was due to
   (a) Blast of rice (b) Brown spot of rice
   (c) Bacterial blight of rice (d) Rice tungro
9. Irish famine of 1845 was due to
   (a) Early blight of potato b) Brown spot of rice
   (c) Bacterial blight of rice (d) Late bligtht of potato
10. Rust disease includes in–
   (a) Deuteromycotina (b) Basidiomycotina
   (c) Ascomycotina (d) Oomycetes

Answer

Q. No.	Answer	Q. No.	Answer
1	(a) Disease	6	(b) B.B. Mundkur
2	(d)All	7	All
3	(c) Abiotic agents	8	(b) Brown spot of rice
4	(a) Continnuous irritation	9	(d) Late bligtht of potato
5	(b) Discontinuous irritation	10	(b) Basidiomycotina

b.True /False

1. Disease as not a pathogen.
2. Disease is a symptom.
3. Disease is not a condition as the condition results from disease and is not synonymous with it.
4. Disease is not an injury.
5. Disease cannot be infectious, it is actually the pathogen which is infectious.

6. Disease results from continuous irritation.
7. Disease is a pathological process.
8. Plant diseases may limit the kinds of plants and industries in the area.
9. Injuries occur when plants are temporarily disturbed.
10. Coffee rust happen in Srilanka in seventees.

Q. No.	Answer	Q. No.	Answer
1	True	6	True
2	False	7	True
3	True	8	True
4	True	9	True
5	True	10	True

B. Descriptive Questions

a. Short Answer

1. Which pathogens do not satisfy Koch's postulates and why?
2. Describe the socio-economic impacts of plant diseases.
3. Write down the difference between disease *and* injury.
4. Define disease and its importance.
5. Mention the importance of plant disease in agriculture.

b. Long Answer

1. What is disease? Mention importance of plant disease in agriculture with suitable classical examples.
2. Differentiate between the healthy (normal) and the diseased plant.
3. Disdinguish between I. Science and art of plant pathology II.Disease and injury III. Disease and disorder IV. Soil invaders and Soil inhabitant.
4. Mention two important milestones in the development of the subject of plant pathology.
5. Mention five plant disease outbreaks with significant effects in more recent times on human civilization.
6. Expalin old and new concept of disease in plants

3

Different Terms used in Plant Pathology

For the accurate identification and diagnosis of plant disease and plant problems a foundational knowledge of terms and definitions is vital for developing concepts, doing research, discussing and communicating issues and providing clarity to your work. The following terms and definitions are basic to the study of plant pathology. They are, however, just a brief introduction to the vocabulary of the science. If you have limited or no background in the subject and you are just getting started, the concepts and terminology of plant problems can seem somewhat daunting. However, your vocabulary and skill will develop through exposure to diagnostics, experience and correct use of the appropriate terms.

Plant pathology (gr., path -"suffering"- "logy", the science of) is the study of plant diseases and the abnormal conditions that constitute plant disorders. **Etiology** is the determination and study of the cause of disease. A pathogen can be living or non-living, but usually refers to a live agent. A **pathogen** is an organism which causes a disease. **Pathological** is a condition of being diseased. **Pathogenic** is having the characteristics of a pathogen and **pathogenicity** is the capability of a pathogen to cause a disease

A plant disease is an abnormality in the structure and/or function of the host plant cells and/or tissue as a result of a continuous irritation caused by a pathogenic agent or an environmental factor. A disease is not static; it is a series of changes in the plant. All plants, to some extent, are subject to disease. Plant disease is the result of an infectious, or biotic (a living component of an ecosystem) agent or a noninfectious, abiotic (non living, physical and/ or chemical component) factor. **Plant injury** is an abrupt alteration of form or function caused by a discontinuous irritant. Plant injury includes insect, animal, physical, chemical or environmental agents.

A causal agent is a general term used to describe an animate or inanimate factor which incites and governs disease and injury. A **causal organism** is a pathogen of biotic origin. When a pathogenic agent is virulent it can cause disease and if the agent is avirulent it is a variant of a pathogen that does not cause severe disease .

A **parasite** is an organism which lives on or in another organism and obtains its nutrition there from. An **obligate parasite** is an organism which is wholly dependent for its nutrition on another living entity. Obligate parasites are **biotrophs** which also depend entirely on a living host for its nutrition. An **autotroph** is a plant that can make its own food through photosynthesis. A **facultative parasites** has the ability, or "faculty" to adapt to an alternative mode of living, saprophytes are organisms that gain their nourishment by digesting dead organic material. Keep in mind that a **parasite** is defined by how the organism secures its nutrients and a **pathogen** is defined on the basis of causing abnormalities. Environmental disease includes such factors as extremes in weather, nutrient deficiency or excess, toxic chemicals and other nonliving agents.

A **host** is an organism (eg. a plant) that is harboring a parasite or pathogen from which it obtains its nutrients. The **host range** refers to the various kinds of host plants that a given pathogen may parasitize. A host is considered **resistant** when it has the ability to exclude, hinder or overcome the effects of a given pathogen or other damaging factor. A plant may be resistant to one pathogen or condition but not others. **Tolerance** is the ability of a plant to be colonized by a pathogen or exposed to an abiotic factor without dying or demonstrating disease symptoms. **Susceptibility** is the antithesis of resistance.

Symbiosis is the mutually beneficial association between two or more different kinds of organisms. The organisms in this association are referred to as **symbionts**. An example of symbiosis is demonstrated in the beneficial relationship between mycorrhizal fungi and the roots of over 85% of the plants in nature. The relationship between mycorrhizal fungi and the host roots of the plant result in increased surface area for absorption of nutrients and water. In return the fungi gain carbohydrates (simple sugars) from the plant. Other examples are the nitrogen-fixing nodules on the roots of legumes caused by bacteria of the genus Rhizobium and the symbiotic relationship of certain fungi and a photosynthetic partner, either an alga or a cyanobacterium, as in lichens.

The **signs** and **symptoms** of plant disorders are the appearance or manifestation of changes in the normal form and/or function of the plant. Signs and symptoms are usually the first indication you will notice in plant problems. **Signs** are the appearance and/or physical evidence of the causal factor of the plants abnormality. **Signs** are the physical evidence of damage caused by biotic or abiotic agents such as the pathogen itself, pests, spores, fruiting bodies, chemical residue, bacterial ooze and so forth. **Symptoms** are the visible response of a plant to biotic and/or abiotic factors that result in a change or abnormality in the plant. Symptoms can take form as galls, chlorosis, ring-spots, wilt, rot and so on. A **syndrome** is the totality of the effects demonstrated in a host by one disease, whether simultaneously or successively, and whether visible to the unaided eye or not. **Diagnostics** is the determination of the nature and/or cause of a disease or disordered condition.

For a biotic disease to occur, the environmental conditions must be conducive to the survival of the pathogen. This is especially true with moisture and temperature. Environmental factors can encourage or discourage the susceptibility of the host and the pathogenicity of the pathogen. The environmental conditions can also effect the interaction between the host and the pathogen. Environmental diseases are caused by persistent unfavorable environmental conditions. These conditions include temperature, moisture, wind, light, soil pH, soil structure, host nutrition, herbicides, chemicals and air pollutants. Nutrient deficiency and excess also can greatly affect the susceptibility of plants to disease and disorders. The four fundamental elements required for disease in plants are: a **susceptible host,** a **pathogen** capable of causing disease, a **favorable environment** and **adequate time**. This is referred to as the **"disease quadrangle"**.

The **life cycle** of an infectious disease is the sequence of distinct events, such as sexual reproduction, that occur between the appearance and reappearance of the causal organism. The stages of the disease cycle are the appearance, development and perpetuation of a pathogen and the effect of the disease on the host. Because advancement of the disease involves the host, the pathogen and in some cases biological vectors, the life cycle of the pathogen as well as environmental factors are involved in the disease cycle. **Propagules** are any structure, fragment or part of an organism that can propagate the organism. The propagules, such as spores, sclerotia etc. that overwinter or oversummer and initiate an infection are referred to as **primary inoculum**. **Secondary inoculum** is produced by infections that take place during the same growing season. **Inoculation** is the process of applying inoculum to a host. Inoculum must be on a part of the host that can be invaded, this is the **infection court**. A **repeating cycle** is a series of secondary infections that continue for a specific period of time during the growing season. A **polycyclic** disease is one that completes two or more life cycles in one year. A **monocyclic** disease is one that has one life cycle in one year.

Pathogens are transmitted, disseminated and spread by many factors, which include biotic, abiotic and environmental factors. **Transmission** usually implies active transfer by means of grafting, insects, mechanical factors, animals and so on. To disseminate or spread means to disperse or distribute. **Disseminate** usually refers to long-distance distribution, and spread usually refers to local distribution. **Vectors** are active agents of transmission such as insects, mites, nematodes and other animals. The dissemination of pathogenic organisms can also be accomplished by wind, rain, irrigation, contaminated seeds and transplants. A few pathogens have the ability to move short distances on their own. Nematodes, zoosporic fungi, oomycetes and some bacteria can move from host to host if they are close enough to one another and the conditions are favorable.

Infection is the establishment of a parasite on or within a host cell or tissue. The **infection court** is a certain part of a given plant that is susceptible to a particular pathogen or pathogens. Successful infections usually result in the appearance of disease symptoms. **Colonization** of a host results from the establishment, growth and reproduction of the pathogen on or in infected plant. **Infestation** refers to the establishment (or "running over") on the surface of a host by a large number of insects or other animal pests. With infestation there is no implication that infection has occurred.

An **epidemic** is the unarrested, widespread increase of an infectious disease, usually limited in time. An epidemic may extend over a single season or many years and over a wide or relatively small area. An **endemic** disease is one that is permanently established in a moderate or severe form within a defined area. Endemic diseases usually become indigenous following initial introduction of the pathogen. **Epidemiology** is the study of factors affecting the outbreak and spread of infectious disease. The **epidemic rate** is the increase or decrease per unit or time in a given plant population.

The classification of a disease can be categorized by the pathogen, the host, the age of the host, the name of the disease, a plant part, symptoms, location, causal agent, geography or by order of importance within a given location. **Taxonomic classification** is the systematic ordering of plants and animals.

There is a very impressive and extensive number of terms and definitions used in plant science, many of which you will not come in contact with. With interest, study and practice, terms and names will come to light and become familiar to you. When you start out, don't worry too much about the scientific names of pathogens and diseases; but also don't be afraid of them. The more exposure you have to the subject the more comfortable you will be when dealing with your peers and the public. In time you will start to notice patterns in both nomenclature and in the biology of pathogens and diseases. These patterns will give you an overall appreciation of this science and a foundational knowledge on which to build your expertise. The feeling of being overwhelmed with new information is a common theme among all of us

Model Practice Questions

A. Objective Questions

a. Multiple Choice Questions

1. An abnormality in the structure and/or function of the host plant cells and/ or tissue as a result of a continuous irritation caused by a pathogenic agent or an environmental factor

   (a) Disease (b) Disorder

   (c) Pathology (d) Pathogen

2. Capability of a pathogen to cause a disease

   (a) Pathogenicity (b) Pathogenesis

   (c) Virulence (d) Avirulence

3. Chain of events leading to the development of the disease

   (a) Pathogenicity (b) Pathogenesis

   (c) Virulence (d) All

4. Degree of pathogenicity is

   (a) Pathogenicity (b) Pathogenesis

   (c) Virulence (d) All

5. Organism which lives on or in another organism and obtains its nutrition there from

   (a) Parasite (b) Saprophyte

   (c) Symbiont (d) Mutualism

6. An organism that is ordinarily saprophytic but under proper conditions may be parasitic.

   (a) Obligate Parasite (b) Obligate Saprophyte

   (c) Facultative Parasite (b) Facultative Saprophyte

7. Physical evidence of disease caused by biotic or abiotic agents

   (a) Sign (b) Symptom

   (c) Syndrome (d) All

8. Totality of the effects demonstrated in a host by one disease, whether simultaneously or successively, and whether visible to the unaided eye or not

   (a) Sign (b) Symptom

   (c) Syndrome (d) All

9. The process of applying inoculums to a host
   (a) Inoculation (b) Infection
   (c) Incubation (d) Dissemination
10. The establishment of host parasitic relationship is called
   (a) Inoculation (b) Infection
   (c) Incubation (d) Dissemination
11. Disease is one that completes two or more life cycles in one year
   (a) Poycyclic disease (b) Monocyclic disease
   (c) Polyetic disease (d) All
12. Disease is one that completes one life cycle in one year
   (a) Poycyclic disease (b) Monocyclic disease
   (c) Polyetic disease (d) All
13. Organism which entirely depends on a living host for its nutrition
   (a) Obligate Parasite (b) Obligate Saprophyte
   (c) Facultative Parasite (b) Facultative Saprophyte
14. The periodically and widespread increase of an infectious disease, usually limited in time
   (a) Epidemic (b) Endemic
   (c) Pandemic (b) Sporadic
15. The disease is one that is permanently established in a moderate or severe form within a defined area.
   (a) Epidemic (b) Endemic
   (c) Pandemic (b) Sporadic

Answer

Q. No	Answer	Q. No	Answer
1	(a) Disease	7	(a) Sign
2	(a) Pathogenicity	8	(c) Syndrome
3	(b) Pathogenesis	9	(a) Inoculation
4	(c) Virulence	10	(b) Infection
5	(a) Parasite	11	(a) Poycyclic disease
6	(c) Facultative parasite	12	(b) Monocyclic disease
13	(a) Obligate parasite	14	(a) Epidemic
15	(b) Endemic		

b.True /False

1. Facultative saprophyte is an organism that is ordinarily parasitic but under proper conditions may be saprophytic.
2. Pathogens are transmitted, disseminated and spread by many factors, which include biotic, abiotic and environmental factors.
3. Transmission usually implies active transfer by means of grafting, insects, mechanical factors, animals etc.
4. Disseminate usually refers to long-distance distribution.
5. Spread usually refers to local distribution.
6. Vectors are active agents of transmission.
7. The infection court is a certain part of a given plant that is susceptible to a particular pathogen or pathogens.
8. Colonization of a host results from the establishment, growth and reproduction of the pathogen on or in infected plant.
9. Propagules are any structure, fragment or part of an organism that can propagate the organism.
10. The epidemic rate is the increase or decrease per unit or time in a given plant population.

Q. No	Answer	Q. No	Answer
1	True	6	True
2	False	7	True
3	True	8	True
4	True	9	True
5	True	10	True

B. Descriptive Questions

a. Short answer questions

1. Define virulence and aggresiveness.
2. Differentiate between obligate and facultative parasite.
3. Define infection and infestation.
4. Define etiology and diagnosis.
5. Differentiate between polycyclic and polyetic disease.
6. Distinguish between I. monocyclic and polycyclic pathogen II. disease cycle and life cycle III. pandemic and sporadic IV. soil invaders and soil inhabitant.

b. Long answer questions

1. What is pathogenicity in plant pathology, and how does it differ from virulence?
2. Explain the concept of plant resistance to diseases, and the different types of resistance mechanisms that plants utilize.
3. What is the role of phytotoxins in plant-pathogen interactions, and how do they contribute to disease development?
4. What is the difference between biotic and abiotic plant stresses, and how can biotic stresses lead to disease outbreaks?
5. How do fungal pathogens infect plants, and what are the key differences between obligate and facultative pathogens in terms of their infection strategies?
6. What are nematodes, and what role do they play in plant diseases?
7. Describe the process of disease cycle in plant pathogens and its importance in disease management strategies.
8. What is the significance of host specificity in plant-pathogen interactions?
9. How do plant diseases impact global food security, and what strategies can be implemented to minimize these impacts?
10. What is the role of molecular techniques in diagnosing and controlling plant diseases?

4

History of Plant Pathology

History in general reveals chronological account of important events, contribution of persons who significantly influenced the thinking of their era and the interpretations of the observed facts or phenomenon over the period of time. The progress in plant pathology leading to the major land mark in mycology, plant bacteriology, plant virology and plant disease control has been described in chronological order for easy and better understanding of the student in following sub-headings.

Mycology

Year	Contributor (s)	Description
1500	Surapal	Wrote 'Vraksha Ayurveda', the first book in which plant diseases were discussed.
1665	Robert Hook	First observed Teliospore of *Pharagmidium disciflorum* under microscope.
1676	Anton von Leeuwenhoek	Developed the first microscope.
1729	PA Michaeli	Studied fungi and saw their spores on the pieces of water melon . Wrote '*Nova Plantarum Genera'* Known as Father of Mycology.
1743	John Needham	Reported plant parasitic nematodes in wheat galls.
1755	M Tillet	Demonstrated that the bunt of wheat was contagious thought that the spores contained a poisonous entity.
1807	B.Prevost	Proofed the role of a micro organism in the causation of disease. Demonstrated the control of wheat smut by steeping seed in copper sulphate solution.
1821	E.M.Fries	Reported that smut and rust fungi as product of diseased plants. Wrote " Systema Mycologium" Known as Linnaeus of Mycology.
1827	Cragie	Showed function of Puccinia in rust fungi.
1840	LR Tulasne & C Tulasne	Confirmed the observation of Prevost with regard to the causal organism of wheat bunt. Known as Reconstructor of Mycology.
1858	JG Kuhn	Published first text book on Plant Pathology namely "The Diseases of Cultivated Crops: Their Causes and Their Control"

Year	Contributor (s)	Description
1861-65	Anton de Bary	First to indicate the nature of obligate and facultative forms. Proved the real cause of late blight of potato is *Phytophthroa infestans*. Described the sex and account of development in number of Phycomyetes and Ascomycetes. Described the role of enzymes in tissue disintegration wile working on soft rot of carrots caused by *Sclerotinia* spp. Demontrated heterocious nature of stem rust of wheat.
1875	O Brefeld	Developed pure culture technique.
1878	M. S. Woronin	Found out the life cycle of potato wart disease.
1881	HM Ward	Reporeted the role of environment in the epidemiology of coffee rust. Father of Tropical Plant Pathology
1882	Robert Hartig	Published a textbook -Diseases of Trees. He is called as "Father of Forest Pathology".
1885	PM Millardet	Discovered the Bordeaux mixture for the control of downey mildew of grapes.
1885	Frank	Discovered Mycorrhizal fungi.
1887	Mason	Introduced Burgundy mixture.
1887	Jensen	Developed hot water technique for wheat smut.
1894	Ericsson	Reported Physiological specialization in stem rust of wheat.
1904	AF Blakeslee	Founded heterothallism in *Rhizopus*.
1904	RH Biffen	First to show that resistance to pathogens in plants can be inheritedas a Mendelian character
1905	RH Biffen	Demonstrated inheritance of rust resistance in wheat in a Medelain fashion.
1917	EC Stakman	Distinguished biological forms in cereal rusts.
1923	Hansen and Smith	Term Heterokaryosis.
1931	PA Saccardo	Wrote "Syllogue Fungorum".
1931	JC Luthra	Solar heat treatment for loose smut of wheat.
1946	HH Flor	Gave gene for gene hypothesis while working on linseed rust.
1952	G Pontecorvo and JA Roper	Discovered parasexuality in *Aspergillus nidulans*.
1968	Vander Plank	Concept of horizontal and vertical resistance. Father of Plant Epidemiology.
1990	DF Klessig and I Raskin; JP Metraux and J Tyals	Demonstrated that salicylic acid is associated with systemic acquired resistance.
2005	RA Dean and Co-workers	The first complete genome sequencing of a plant pathogenic fungus *Magnaporthe grisea*.

Plant Bacteriology

Year	Contributor (s)	Description
1683	Anton von Leeuwenhoek	First observed bacteria.
1876	Robert Koch	They proved that anthrax disease of cattle was caused by specific bacterium.
1876	Louis Pasteur	Demonstrated role of bacteria in fermentation and decay.
1876	Robert Koch	Described the theory called "Koch's postulates." He established the principles of pure culture technique.
1876	Robert Koch and Pasteur	Disproved the theory of spontaneous generation of diseases and propose germ theory in relation to the diseases of man and animal.
1876	Woronin	Isolated and described the root nodule bacteria in leguminous plant.
1878	TJ Burril	Described first bacterial disease (Fire blight of apples) caused by *Erwinia amylovora.*
1879.	Prilleaux	Reported the bacterial decay of wheat kernels.
1883	JH Wakker	Investigated yellow slime disease of hyacinth caused by bacterium.
1885-1887	JC Arther	Confirmed Burrill's work.
1887	EF Smith	Gave the final proof that bacteria could be the incitants of plant diseases. First to notice and study the crown gall disease. Father of Phytobacteriology.
1980	DW Dye and Co-workers	Introduced pathovar system in taxonomy.
1910	CO Jensen	Related crown gall of plants to cancer of animals.
1952	J. Lederberg	Coined the term plasmid.
1952	SA Waksman	Discovered streptomycin.
1952	Zinder and J. Lederberg	Discovered transduction in bacteria.
1962	H Stolp	Discovered bdellovibrios.
1972	PB New and A Kerr	Success in biological control of *A. radiobacter* strain K.
1972	IM Windsor and LM Black	Observed a new kind of phloem inhabiting bacterium causing clover club leaf disease.
1972	Windsor and Black	Observed rickettsia like organisms in the phloem of clover plants infected with the club leaf disease.
1974	I Zanen et al	Demonstrated Ti plasmid in *Agrobacterium tumefaciens.*
1977	Chilton et al.	Showed that the crown gall bacterium transforms normal plant cells into tumor cells by introducing into them a plasmid, part of which becomes inserted into the plant cell chromosomes DNA.

Plant Virology

Year	Contributor (s)	Description.
1576	C Clusius	Recorded Breaking of tulips owing to viral infection.
1857.	Swietch	Identified Tobacco mosaic.
1886	AE Mayer	First to point out that tobacco mosaic is readily transmissible and infectious. Demonstrated the sap transmission of the TMV.
1892	D Ivanowski	Demonsrated that the agents of TMV could pass through filters that retained bacterial cells (bacteria proof filter).
1894	Hashimoto	Showed transmissiblelity of rice dwarf disease by leaf hopper (*Nephotettix apicalis var. cincticeps*).
1898	MW Beijernick	Concept of contagium vivum fluidum Father of Plant Virology.
1917	d'Herelle	Discovered bacteriophage.
1932	Knoll and Ruska	Invented Electron microscope.
1935	WM Stanley	Crystallized Tobacco mosaic virus.
1936	Bawden and NW Pirie	Found that the crystalline nature of the virus contains nucleic acid and protein.
1939	Kausche, Pfankuch and Ruska	Saw virus particles for the first time with the electron microscope. Confirmed that TMV was rod shaped.
1942 & 1944	Muller Williams and Wycoff	Developed shadow casting technique with heavy metals which was useful for determining the overall size and shape of the virus particles.
1949	Markham and Smith	Isolated TYMV and showed that it contained (1) An infectious nucleoprotein (about 25%) and (2) non inferious protein.
1952	Morel and Martin	Showed that virus free plants could be obtained from totally infected parents using meristem tip culture.
1954	Kassanis	Showed that virus could be eradicated from infected plants by high temperature treatment.
1956	Gierer and Schramm	Proved that the nucleic acid fraction of the virus is actually the infectious agent.
1966.	Kassanis	Discovered the satellite viruses.
1963 & 1966	Black and Markhan; Miura et al	Showed that wound tamout and rice dwarf viruses contain double started RNA.
1967	Doi and Co-workers	Discovered Mycoplasma like organism
1967	Ishiie et al	showed that the MLO bodies and the symptoms disappeared temporarily when the plants were treated with tetracycline antibodies.
1967	Diener and Raymer	Discovered viroid
1968	Shephard et al	Showed that cauliflower mosaic virus contains double stranded DNA.
1974	Davies &Worley	Coined the term spiroplasma.

1977	Clark and Adams	Develpoed ELISA assay for detection of plant viruses.
1981	TW Randles and | co-workers	Discovered virusoids.
1982	Prusiner	Discovered Prions
1994	Sears and Krikpatrick	MLO that infects plants have been reclassified as Phytoplasmas.

Plant Disease Control

Year	Contributor (s)	Description
1000	Homer	Mentioned about the use of sulphur in plant disease control.
1807	B Prevost	Recommended copper sulphate for wheat seed treatment against bunt and demonstrated first time the fungitoxic value of copper compounds.
1882	PMA Millardet	Discovered Bordeaux mixture for control of downy mildew of grape vine.
1887	Mason	Discovered burgundy mixture.
1921	Bewley	Developed chestnut compound.
1934	Tisdale and Williams	Reported fungitoxicity of dithiocarbamates.
1942	Singh	Delveloped Chaubatia paste.
1943	SA Waksman and A Schatx	Discovered Streptomycin.
1952	Kittleson	Discovered captan also known as Kittleson's Killer.
1966	Von Schmeling and M Kulka	Discovered Systemic fungicides oxanthin.

Plant Pathology in India

Year	Contributor (s)	Description
1885	KR Kritikar	First Indian scientist who collected and identified fungi.
1886-1971	JF Dastur	First Indian Plant pathologistknown for the establishment of genus Phytophthora and diseases caused by it in castor and potato.
	TS Sadasivan	Developed concept of vivotoxins and worked out the mechanism of wilting in cotton owing to *Fusarium oxysporum* f. sp. *vasinfectum*.
	SN Dasgupta	Carried out exensive study on black tip of mango.
	MJ Thrimalachar	Discovered several antifungal antibiotics viz aureofungin, haymycin etc.
	YL Nene	Reported Khaira disease of rice caused due to Zn deficiency Authored book "*Fungicides in Plant Disease Control*".
1889	DD Cunningham	Reported the causal organism of red rust of tea in Assam caused by *Cephaleurous virescens.*

1920	EJ Butler	First direcotor of Imperial Mycological Institue in England. Initiated an exhaustive study on Indian fungi and the disease caused by them Discovered genus Allomyces. Wrote "*Fungi and Diseases in Plants*" Father of Indian Plant Pathology.
1940	KC Mehta	Studied epidemiology of cereal rusts in India Write monograph on "*Further studies on cereal rust in India*" *Father of Indian Rust.*
1948	BB Mundukar	Established Indian Phytopathological society with its journal "*Indian Phytopathology*".
1953	JC Luthra and A Sattar	Developed solar heat treatment for loose smut of wheat.
	Ramanujam and Co-workers	Developed seed plot technique for virus free seed potato production in Indo Gangetic plains.
1975	S Nagrajan and H Singh	Formulated Indian Stem Rust Rules for *Puccinia graminis tritici.*

Model Question Papers

A. Objective Questions

a. Multiple choice Questions

1. Who reported that virus can be crystallized and still retain infectivity
   - (a) Adolf Mayer (b) D Ivanowski
   - (c) M. Beijerinck (d) W Staley
2. Who reported that complete infectious TMV particle can be reconstituted *in vitro* from the RNA and protein component
   - (a) Adolf Mayer (b) D Ivanowski
   - (c) Fraenkel –Conrat (d) W Staley
3. Who among the following completely sequenced potato spindle tuber viroid
   - (a) Heinz Sanger (b) Bawden &Pirie
   - (c) Fraenkel –Conrat (d) W Staley
4. Who disproves the theory of Spontaneous generation –
   - (a) Heinz Sanger (b) Bowden &Pirie
   - (c) L. Spallanzani (d) Louis Pasteur
5. Who invented PCR
   - (a) Karry Mullis (b) Peter Perlmann
   - (c) Stanley (d) Ev Engavall

6. Who developed NA hybridization technique for identification of viroid
   (a) Karry Mullis (b) Peter Perlmann
   (c) Randles *et al* (d) Ev Engavall
7. In 2005 which pathological scientist got Borlaug award–
   (a) Rattan Lal (b) VL Chopra
   (c) CD Mayee (d) S Nagarajan
8. Renowned scientist Dr. N.E. Borlaug belongs to–
   (a) Agronomy (b) Genetics
   (c) Entomology (d) Plant Pathology
9. Who did most of his work on rust diseases in India–
   (a) R Prasad (b) KC Mehta
   (c) BB Mundakur (d) EJ Butler
10. Who is the father of American Nematology ?
   (a) JG Kuhn (b) H Schacht
   (c) NA Cobb (d) T J Burill
11. The term virus was first time coined by
   (a) Kuhn (b) Beijerinck
   (c) Stanley (d) None of these
12. Father of Indian Mycology–
   (a) EJ Butler (b) KC Mehta
   (c) BB Mundakur (d) RS Singh
13. Significant contribution on the epidemiology of disease cycle of stem rust of wheat was made by
   (a) KC Mehta (b) BB Mundkur
   (c) MM Payak (d) S Nagarajan
14. The Indian Phytopathological society was started by
   (a) B.B.Mundkur (b) Coleman
   (c) E.J.Butler (d) Kirtikar
15. Who advanced the gene for gene concept of disease and resistance and susceptibility
   (a) Biffen and Orton (b) H H Flor
   (c) Vander plank (d) Gaumann

16. The term Virus was coined by
    (a) Adolf Meyer (b) Stanley
    (c) Beijerinck (d) Ivanowski
17. Parasexuality in fungi was first discovered by
    (a) Pontecarvo &Roper (b) Erickson
    (c) Anton de Bary (d) Robert Koch
18. The systemic fungicide oxanthin was discovered by
    (a) Vanderplank (b) Kittleson
    (c) Von Schmelling & Kulka (d) Tisdale and Williams
19. Renowned scientist Dr. N.E. Borlaug belongs to
    (a) Agronomy (b) Genetics
    (c) Entomology (d) Plant Pathology
20. Who demonsrated that the agents of TMV could pass through filters that retained bacterial cells
    (a) Adolf Meyer (b) Stanley
    (c) Beijerinck (d) Ivanowski

Q. No	Answer	Q. No	Answer
1	(d) W Staley	11	(b) Beijerinck
2	(c) Fraenkel –Conrat	12	(a) E.J. Butler
3	(a) Heinz Sanger	13	(a) Mehta. K.C
4	(d) Louis Pasteur	14	(a) B.B.Mundkur
5	(a) Karry Mullis	15	(b) H H Flor
6	(c) Randles *et al*	16	(c) Beijerinck
7	(d) S Nagarajan	17	(a) Pontecarvo &Roper
8	(d) Plant Pathology	18	(c) Von Schmelling & Kulka
9	(b) KC Mehta	19	(d) Plant Pathology
10	(c) NA Cobb	20	(d) Ivanowski

b. True/False

1. Robert Koch established that a particular bacterium was the source of the cattle anthrax disease.
2. Burril TJ first bacterial disease to be described, *Erwinia amylovora*-caused fire blight on apples
3. EF Smith is regarded as the father of phytobacteriology.
4. Zinder and J. Lederberg discovered the bacterial transduction mechanism.
5. Contagium vivum fluidum theory was introduced by MW Beijernick.

6. The green ear or downy mildew of pearlmillet was first time reported in India by E J Butler.
7. The oxathiin fungicide was first time discovered by Yon Schmeling and Kulka.
8. Kamal bunt of wheat first time reported in Karnal by Mitra .
9. NA Cobb is known as the father of American Nematology .
10. YL Nene reported rice Khaira disease caused on by a zinc deficiency.
11. *Puccinia graminis tritici's* Indian Stem Rust Rules were developed by S Nagrajan and H Singh.
12. MJ Thrimalachar discovered various antifungal antibiotics, such as haymycin and aureofungin.
13. B. Prevost suggested using copper sulfate to treat wheat seeds against bunt and proving for the first time the fungitoxic potential of copper compounds.
14. Doi and colleagues discovered an organism like Mycoplasma.
15. K.C.Mehta wrote a monograph on "Further studies on cereal rust in India"

Q. No.	Answer	Q. No	Answer
1	True	9	True
2	True	10	True
3	True	11	True
4	True	12	True
5	True	13	True
6	True	14	True
7	True	15	True
8	True	16	-

B. Descriptive Questions

a. Short answers

1. Write an essay on history of Plant Pathology ?
2. Name two ancient Indian holy books in which reference to plant diseases and their control devices is made.
3. What would have been the main reason, in your opinion, behind they very slow growth of plant pathology upto the time of Antony Van Leeuwenhoek?
4. Who is credited to have laid the foundation of the "science" of plant pathology? How?

5. Name the authors of the books "Fungi and Diseases in Plants" and "Fungi and Plant Diseases".
6. What were the conclusions made by Ivanowski (1882) and Beijerinck (1898) in reference to the experiments on tobacco mosaic disease?

b. Long answer

1. Write an essay on developments of various disciplines of plant pathology upto 19th century.
2. Give a concise account of the main Indian contributions in plant pathology.
3. Write notes on:
   a. Discovery of Bordeaux mixture.
   b. Adolf Mayer's contribution in development of virology.
   c. Germ theory of disease.
   d. Multidisciplinary nature of plant pathology.
4. Mention the most important contributions of the following Indian Plant Pathologists. i.K.C. Mehta ii.B.B.Mundkar iii.M.J.Thirumalachar iv.G.S.Kulkarni .
5. Name five contemporary scientists of Plant Pathology in India.

5

Causes of Plant Disease

Plant diseases are classified on the basis of type of pathogenic or non-pathogenic causes of the disease. The classification is based on the plant pathogenic organisms as follows.

1. Parasites

They include both biotic and mesobiotic agents. The diseases are incited by parasites under a set of suitable environment. Association of definite pathogen is essential with each disease.

i. Biotic agents: They are also called as animate causes. They are living organisms.Biotic agents include

1. Prokaryotes

a. True bacteria or bacteria (Facultative parasites) e.g. Citrus canker.

b. Rickettsia-like bacteria (RLB) e.g. Citrus greening, Pierce's disease of grape.

c. Mollicutes or wall-less prokaryotes

  i. Mycoplasma-like organism (MLO) e.g. Sesame phyllody, Egg plant little leaf.

  ii. Spiroplasma e.g. Corn stunt, Citrus stubborn.

2. Eukaryotes

a. Protists (Unicellular, coenocytic or multicellular with little or no differentiation of cells and tissues).

  i. Fungi e.g. wilt of cotton

  ii. Protozoa e.g. heart rot of coconut

  iii. Algae e.g. red rust of mango

b. Plants - Parasitic flowering plants or phanerogamic parasites - Broomrape of tobacco etc.

c. Animals- Nematodes –Root knot nematode etc.

Mesobiotic agents: They include viruses and viroids. They are infectious agents. They can be crystallized and are considered non-living. But their multiplication in the living plants ensures that they are living. Hence they are called as mesobiotic agents.

a. Viruses e.g. Yellow mosaic of blackgram

b. Viroids e.g. Spindle tuber of potato

2. Non-parasites or Abiotic agents or Physiological disorders

Definition

Plant disease in which no pathogens or parasitic is associate with the cause is known as **Non-parasitic** disease. They are also called as **non-infectious** or **physiological disorders**. When no pathogen is found, cultured from or transmitted from a diseased plant, then the disease is said to be caused by a non-living or environmental factor. These diseases occur because of disturbances in the plant system by the improper environmental conditions in the air or soil or by mechanical influences. .

General Characteristics

1. Physiological disease occurs in the absence of pathogen and therefore, cannot be transmitted.
2. Physiological disorder of plants is caused by the lack or excess of something that supports life from diseased to healthy plants.
3. Non infectious disease may effect plant in all stages of their lives, such as seeds, seedlings, mature plants or fruits.
4. Symptoms may range from slight to severe and affected plants may even die.
5. These disease cause damage in field in storage or at the market.

Factors responsible for physiological disorder or Non parasitic disease

1. Unfavourable temperature

i) Effects of low temperature

1. Low temperature causes greater damage to crops than high temperature.
2. The frost injuries involved killing of buds of peach, cherry, killing of flowers, young fruits and sometimes succulent twings of most trees.
3. Blotch type necrosis in potato is due to freezing injury.
4. Low winter temperature may kill young roots of trees such as apple and may also cause canker development. and bark splitting.

ii) Effects of high temperature

1. Plants are normally injured quicker and to a greater extent when temperature becomes higher than maximum for growth.
2. High temperature are by and large responsible for sun scald injuries appearing the sun exposed sides of fleshy fruits and vegetables. For example. Sun scald of apple, tomato, onion- bulbs, peppers, potato tubers, canker of linseeds.

2. Effects of moisture

i). Effects of low moisture

Plant suffering from lack or sufficient soil moisture generally remain stunted are pale green to light yellow, have hardly any small dropping leaves and finally in absence of moisture plant dry and wilt.

ii). Effects of high moisture

Excessive moisture by flooding in the field may cause decay or rotting of fibrous root of plants resulting into wilting. Primarily due to accumulation of toxic materials around the root and base of stem and also due to non availability of nutrients. For example. Tip burn of paddy.

3. Inadequate Oxygen

When there is too much respiration in closed atmosphere the entire oxygen supply may be exhausted resulting in disintegration of cells due to enzymic action. For example. Black heart of potato.

4. Unfavourable Light

Absence of light or lack of sufficient light retards chlorophyll formation and promotes slender growths with long internodes, thus leading to pale green leaves, spirally growth and premature drop of leaves and flower. This condition is known as "**Etiloation**".

5. Atmospheric Impurities

Presence of injurious gases in the atmosphere may cause definite injury to plant and plant parts. More severe and wide spread damage is caused to plant in the fields by chemicals such as hydrogen fluoride, nitrogen dioxide, ozone, sulphur dioxide, peroxyaacotyl nitrates. For example. Black tip of mango . Fruit on trees in close proximity to brick kilns may bear necrotic lesions and become useless for sale and consumption The smoke of kills polluted the air with toxic gases like sulphur dioxide which caused necrosis of tissues.

6. Soil mineral toxicity and toxic effects of decomposition of organic matter in soil

Excessive amount of sodium salt especially sodium sulphate, sodium chloride, and sodium carbonate raise the PH of the soil and cause alkali injury i.e chlorosis, stunting etc. Boron, copper and manganese have been most often implicated in mineral toxicity disease. Excess manganese is known to cause crinkle leaf disease in cotton. Excess boron is toxic to many vegetable and trees.

Crop residue decomposing in soil produce toxic substances such as fatty acids which produce symptoms of damping off, root rot, wilt and nutritional deficiency.

7. Herbicidal Injury

Several of the most common plant disorder seems to be the result of extensive use of herbicides. Increasing number of herbicides in use for general or specific weed control has created problems.

8. Nutritional Deficiencies or Disorder in Plants

i) Deficiency of minerals *viz*, nitrogen, phosphorus, potash, manganese , zinc, copper , iron, magnesium, boron, , etc. results in disorders in plant metabolism and cause hunger signs in the crops.

ii) Excess of minerals disturbs nutritional balance needed for good metabolism in the plant, hence hindering the effect of essential element.

iii) The deficiencies and excess of minerals also reduce the resistance of plant to fungal, bacterial and other diseases.

iv) The kind of symptoms produced by deficiency of a certain nutrient depend primarily on the functions of that particular element in the plant.

Plant disease due to lack of minerals

Sr.No	Deficient Nutrient	Disease
1.	Nitrogen (N)	Red leaf of cotton
2.	Phosphorus (P)	Dwarfening of cotton
3.	Potassium (K)	Cotton rust, leaf spot of alfa alfa.
4.	Magnesium (Mg)	Sand drown disease in tobacco
5.	Boron (B)	Internal cork of apple Cracked stem of celery Black tip of mango Heart rot of sugarbeet Brown heart of cabbage and turnip Internal brown spot of sweet potato Terminal bud breakdown of tobacco Fruit pitting and dieback of olive Hollow stem of brassica

6	Copper (Cu)	Reclamation disease of oats Diebacks of citrus Wither tip of apple
7	Manganese (Mn)	Pahala blight of sugarcane Marsh spot of garden pea Grey speck of oats.
8	Zinc (Zn)	White bud of corn, Little leaf of apple, Bronzing of twigs, Rosette of fruits trees, Mottle leaf of citrus Khaira disease of rice
9	Iron (Fe)	Green netting of citrus
10	Molybdenum (Mo)	Whiptail disease of cauliflower.
11	Calcium (Ca)	Blossom end rot of tomato Black heart of celery Wither tip of flax

Comparison between different plant pathogens

Features	Fungi	Bacteria	**Viruses**	**Viroids**	**Phyto-plasma**	**Sprioplas-ma**	**RLO**	**Protozoa**	**Algae**	**Nematode**
Visibility in micorscope	Yes	Yes	No (visible under Elec-tronmicro-scope)	No (visible under Electron microscope)	Yes	Yes	Yes	Yes	Yes	Yes
Prokaryote / Eukaryote	Eukaryote	Prokaryote	Kingdom -Virus	-	Prokary-ote	Prokaryote	Prokaryote	Eukaryote	Eukary-ote	Eukaryote
Cell Wall	Present	Present	Absent	Absent	Absent	Absent	Present	Present	Present	Present
Cell wall with mucopoly saccharides	No	Yes	Yes	No	No	No	Yes	No	No	No
Nucleic acid	Both DNA & RNA	Both DNA & RNA	Either DNA & RNA	RNA	Both DNA & RNA	Both DNA & RNA	Both DNA & RNA	Both DNA & RNA	Both DNA & RNA	Both DNA & RNA
Protein synthe-sis by their own enzyme	Yes	Yes	No	No	Yes	Yes		Yes	Yes	Yes
Culture in cell free medium	Yes	Yes	Yes	No	No	No	Xylem inhibitory fastidious vascular bacteria can be cultured	Yes	Yes	Yes
Dependent on host nucleic acid for multiplica-tion	No	No		No	No	No	No	No	No	No
Reproduction	Asexual &Sexual	Binary fission	Replication	Replication	Binary fission	Binary fission	Binary fission	Asexual &Sexual	Asexual &Sexual	Asexual &Sexual

Difference between Disease and Disorder

Features	Diasease	Disorder
Symptom expression	Appear progressively at definite stages.	Appear suddenly, nearly all at once in their fullest nature and intensity
Proportion of affected plants in an area	May vary in their extent of disease development	Tend to be affected with similar extent or in a similar way
Symptom variability	Symptoms variable in type, pattern and occurrence, although recognizable other wise	Symtom on individual plant or plant parts are regular or uniform in nature and pattern.
Sign	Present	Absent
Distribution of affected plants	Usually irregular or uneven distribution	Fairly regular or uniform in field or tightly clustered in affected area with no apparent spread pattern.

Difference between Pathogen and Parasite

Features	Pathogen	Parasite
Definition	Any agent that causes damage or disease	Organism existing in an intimate association with another living organisms and derives its nutrition from that host
Plant Pathogen relationship	Most (not all) pathogens are parasites	All parasites are not pathogens
Example	*Ustilago tritici*	Root nodule bacteria (*Rhizobium leguminoserum* on the roots of pulses). Mycorhizal fungus parasitic on roots of trees
Sign	Present	Absent
Distribution of affected plants	Usually irregular or uneven distribution	Fairly regular or uniform in field or tightly clustered in affected area with no apparent spread pattern.

Multiple Choice Questions

A. Objective Questions

a. Multiple Choice Questions

1. Rice blast pathogen perfect stage is–

(a) *Pyricularia oryzae* (b) *Magnaporthe grisea*

(c) *Helmiuthosporium oryzae* (d) *Rhizoctonia solani*

2. Black heart is a physiological disorder of

(a) Tomato (b) Chilli

(c) Potato (d) Cabbage

3. The scientific name of burrowing nematode is–
   (a) *Xiphinema* sp. (b) *Lougidorus* sp.
   (c) *Meloidogyne* sp. (d) *Radopholus similis*.
4. Tea rust is caused by–
   (a) MLO (b) Virus
   (c) Bacteria (d) Algae
5. The major storage fungi that effects the food grain is–
   (a) Rhizobium (b) Mucor
   (c) Cercospora (d) Aspergillus
6. Application of potash increases
   (a) Resistance to water logging (b) Frost resistance in plants
   (c) Disease resistance in plants (d) None of these
7. Viruses contain–
   (a) RNA (b) DNA
   (c) Both RNA and DNA (d) Either RNA or DNA
8. The incidence of black scurf of potato is more in–
   (a) Sandy soil (b) Clay soil
   (c) Alluvial soil (d) Loam soil
9. The causal organism of bunchy top of banana is transmitted by–
   (a) *Pentalonia nigronervosa* (b) *Bemisia tabaci*
   (c) *Lipaphis erisimi* (d) Pollen
10. Mad cow disease is caused by
   (a) Virion (b) Pirion
   (c) Bacteria (d) MLO
11. Black tip of mango is caused due to the deficiency of
   (a) B (b) Zn
   (c) Cu (d) Mo
12. Heart rot of sugarbeet is caused due to the deficiency of
   (a) B (b) Zn
   (c) Cu (d) Mo
13. Khaira disease of rice is caused due to the deficiency of
   (a) B (b) Zn
   (c) Cu (d) Mo

14. Reclamation disease of oats is caused due to the deficiency of

(a) B	(b) Zn
(c) Cu	(d) Mo

15. White bud of corn is caused due to the deficiency of

(a) B	(b) Zn
(c) Cu	(d) Mo

Answer

Q. No	Answer	Q. No.	Answer
1	(b) *Magnaporthe grisea*	6	(c) Disease resistance in plants
2	(c) Potato	7	(d) Either RNA or DNA
3	(a) *Radopholus similis*	8	(a) Sandy soil
4	(d) Algae	9	(a) *Peutalonia nigronervosa*
5	(d) Aspergillus	10	(b) Pirion
11	(a) B	12	(b) Zn
13	(a) B	14	(c) Cu
15	(b) Zn	-	-

b.True /False

1. Sucidal germination takes place in striga.
2. Citrus greening caused by Fastidious bacteria.
3. 'Little leaf' in brinjal is caused by a Mycoplasma.
4. Wither tip of apple is caused due to deficiency of Molybdnum.
5. Pahala blight of Sugarcane is caused due to deficiency of Manganease.
6. The viruses which are usually helped or accompanied by smaller spherical particles of another serologically unrelated virus known as Satellite virus.
7. MLO disease transmitted by Leaf hopper.
8. Green netting of citrus is caused due to deficiency of Iron.
9. Whiptail disease of cauliflower is caused due to deficiency of Molybdnum.
10. Caulimovirus is an example of virus containing ds DNA.
11. Multiplication of virus occurs in Plasmodesmata.
12. Phytoplasmas contain DNA only.
13. NEPO viruses are transmitted by *Xiphinema index.*
14. Blossom end rot of tomato is caused due to deficiency of Calcium.

Q. No	Answer	Q. No.	Answer
1	True	6	True
2	False	7	True
3	True	8	True
4	True	9	True
5	True	10	True
11	True	12	False
13	False	14	True
15	True		

B. Descriptive Questions

a. Short Answer

1. How nutrient mobility determines the site of symptom development?
2. Which elements become deficients in acidic soils?
3. Why is iron not easily available to the plants?
4. Write notes on i. Microbial inoculants, ii.Iron efficient plants iii. Plant disorder caused by Zn. Disorder caused by Fe.
5. Write short notes on i. Disorder caused by B ii. Disorder caused by N iii. Disorder caused by Moiv. Disorder caused by Ca

b. Long Answer Questions

1. What are the biotic, abiotic and mesobiotic pathogens of plant diseases? Give in brief the classification of plant diseases according to major causal agents.
2. Distinguish between biotic and abiotic pathogens .
3. Give two examples each of biotic, abiotic and mesobiotic pathogens.
4. Discuss about physiological disorders in plants.
5. Differentiate between pathogen and parasites.
6. Distinguish between :

   I. Iron efficient and Iron deficient plants

   II. Freezing and Chilling injury

   III. Primary and secondary air pollutants

6

Classification of Plant Diseases

There are thousands of diseases, which attack crop plants. Classification can be made based on several criteria. The various ways of classifying diseases of plants are given below.

A. Based on type of infection

1. **Localized disease**: Affecting only a part of the plant; leaf spots and anthracnoses caused by different fungi.
2. **Systemic disease:** affecting the entire plant.

B. Based on symptoms: Rusts smuts, wilts, blights, cankers, mildews, rots, damping-off, die-back, scab etc.

C. Based on the host plant

1. **On the basis of host** e.g. Diseases of apple, diseases of wheat, diseases of rose, diseases of coconut, diseases of coffee, diseases of cotton.
2. **On the basis of host group**- e.g. cereal crop disease, pulse crop diseases, oilseed crop diseases, root crop disease, forage crop disease, plantation crop disease etc.

D. Based on their occurrence

1. **Endemic disease**: The word endemic means prevalent in, and confined to, a particular country or district and is applied to disease. These diseases are natural to one country or part of the earth. When a disease is more or less constantly present in one form or other or less constantly present form year to year in a moderate to severe form, in a particular country or part of earth, it is classed as endemic.
2. **Epidemic or epiphytotic diseases**: The term 'epidemic' is derived from a Greek word meaning 'among the people' and in true sense applies to those diseases of human beings which appear very virulently among large section of the population. To carry the same sense in the case of plant diseases, the term epiphytotic has been coined. An epiphytotic disease is one which occurs widely but periodically. It may be present constantly in the locality but assumes severe form only on occasions.

3. **Sporadic diseases**: Sporadic diseases are those diseases which occur at very irregular intervals and locations and in relatively few instances. A given disease may be endemic in one region and epidemic in another. When a disease is prevalent throughout the country, continent or the world it is known as a *pandemic* disease.

E. Based on the cause:

1. **Infectious or Biotic disease:** These are diseases which are incited by biotic or mesobiotic agents under a set of suitable environments. Example, fungal disease, bacterial disease, viral disease.
2. **Non-infectious or Abiotic disease**: These are the diseases with no biotic or mesobiotic agents associated, remain noninfectious and cannot be transmitted from one diseased plant to another healthy plant. Example. Disease caused by nature-frost, rain, wind, sun, hail storm et.)

F. Based on the Production of Inoculum

1. **Single cycle disease (Simple Interest Disease):** When the increase of disease is mathematically analogs to simple interest of money, it is called simple interest disease. There is only one generation of disease in the course of one epidemic. Such diseases develop from a common source of inoculums i.e the capital is constant, and often there is one generation of infection in a season. Example. Loose smut of wheat
2. **Multiple cycle Disease (Compound Interest Disease):** When the increase in disease is mathematically analogues to compound interest of money, the disease is called compound interest disease. There are several or many generations of the pathogen in one life cycle of the crop, i.e the capital is increased by the amount of interest. Example. Late blight of potato.

G. Type of perpetuation and spread

1. **Soil-borne diseases**: The causal agents perpetuate and spread through soil. Example. Damping off caused by fungi like *Pythium* sp. and root rot caused by *Rhizoctonia* spp.
2. **Seed-borne diseases**: Seed or seed materials help in the perpetuation and spread of this disease. The disease causing agents may be internally seed-borne or externally seed-borne e.g. Loose smut of wheat caused by *Ustilago nuda tritici* (internally seed borne) and blast of rice caused by *Pyricularia oryzae* (externally seed-borne).
3. **Air-borne diseases**: In these type of diseases the causal agents are spread by wind (air). Example. Early leaf spot and late leaf spot of groundnut

caused by *Cercospora arachidicola* and *Phaeoisariopsis personata* respectively.

H. Based on sugar requirement of the pathogen

Based on the sugar requirements of the pathogen, diseases can be grouped into high sugar diseases or low sugar diseases. Diseases such as rusts and powdery mildews increased when the crops were sprayed with chemicals like DDT or maleic hydrazide which inhibit the outflow of sugars from the leaf and termed these diseases as 'high sugar diseases'. On the other hand when the crops were sprayed with chemicals like 2,4 D which increase the outflow of sugars e.g. the disease like spots increased and termed these diseases as 'low sugar diseases'

I. Iatrogenic diseases

The diseases which appear on the plant while managing major diseases are called iatrogenic diseases e.g. when zineb is sprayed on grapes for the management of downy mildew, the crop suffers losses from grey mold which otherwise do not cause any disease. This happens owing to the effects of the chemical on microclimatic and microbial flora on the leaf surface. The chemical may affect the structural composition or chemical composition of the sugars or the leaf exudates or the phylloplane microflora resulting in conditions favorable for the new pathogen.

Model Practice Questions

A.Objective Questions

a.Multiple Choice Questions

1. When disease affecting only a part of the plant

(a)	Localized disease	(b)	Systemic disease
(c)	Aerial disease	(d)	Endemic disease

2. When disease affecting the entire plant

(a)	Localized disease	(b)	Systemic disease
(c)	Aerial disease	(d)	Endemic disease

3. The term 'epidemic' is derived from a Greek word meaning

(a)	Among the people	(b)	Among the plant
(c)	Among the animal	(d)	Among the insects

4. The term 'epiphytotic ' is derived from a Greek word meaning

(a)	Among the people	(b)	Among the plant
(c)	Among the animal	(d)	Among the insects

5. When a disease is prevalent throughout the country, continent or the world it is known as

   (a) Epidemic (b) Endemic

   (c) Pandemic (b) Sporadic

6. Those diseases which occur at very irregular intervals and locations and in relatively few instances

   (a) Epidemic (b) Endemic

   (c) Pandemic (d) Sporadic

7. 'Low sugar' disease is

   (a) Rust (b) Downy mildew

   (c) Powdery mildew (d) Leaf spot

8 'High sugar' disease is

   (a) Rust (b) Downy mildew

   (c) Powdery mildew (d) All the above

9. The diseases which appear on the plant while managing major diseases are called

   (a) Iatrogenic diseases (b) High sugar disease

   (c) Low sugar disease (d) All

10. The establishment of host parasitic relationship is called

   (a) Inoculation (b) Infection

   (c) Incubation (d) Dissemination

Answer

Q. No	Answer	Q. No	Answer
1	(a) Localized disease	6	(d) Sporadic
2	(b) Systemic disease	7	(d) Leaf spot
3	(a) Among the people	8	(d) All the above
4	(b) Among the plant	9	(a) Iatrogenic diseases
5	(c) Pandemic	10	(b) Infection

b. True/False

1. Damping off caused by fungi is a soil borne disease.
2. Loose smut of wheat is a internally seed borne in nature.
3. The word endemic means prevalent in, and confined to, a particular country or district and is applied to disease.

4. An epiphytotic disease is one which occurs widely but periodically in plant.
5. The term 'endemic' is derived from a Greek word meaning 'among the people.
6. Loose smut of wheat is a cmpound interest disease
7. *Infectious* diseases which are incited by biotic or mesobiotic agents .
8. *Non-infectious* diseases cannot be transmitted from one diseased plant to another healthy plant.
9. Late blight of potato is a simple interest disease.
10. Blast of rice is a externally seed-borne in nature.

Answer

Q. No	Answer	Q. No	Answer
1	True	6	False
2	False	7	True
3	True	8	True
4	True	9	False
5	True	10	True

B. Descriptive Questions

a. Short answer questions

1. Classify disease on the basis of type of infection.
2. Group diseases according to their causes.
3. Classify disease on based on their occurrence.
4. Based on the production of inoculums, categorize diseases.
5. Classify disease based on type of perpetuation and spread.
6. Discuss in details about itragenic diseases.

b. Long answer questions

1. What are the different categories of plant diseases based on their causal agents? Discuss each category in detail with examples.
2. Explain the classification of plant diseases based on symptoms. How are these symptoms used to identify and classify plant diseases? Provide examples of diseases categorized by symptoms.
3. Describe the classification of plant diseases based on their mode of transmission. Discuss the various modes such as airborne, soilborne, and waterborne diseases, and their impact on plant health.

4. What is the significance of classifying plant diseases based on their etiology? Discuss how this classification helps in disease management and control measures.
5. Explain the classification of plant diseases based on the host plant. How are diseases classified according to the plant species they affect? Provide examples of diseases that target specific plants.
6. Discuss the classification of plant diseases based on their environmental conditions. How does climate, soil type, and other environmental factors influence disease development?
7. How are plant diseases classified based on the level of infection? Discuss the differences between primary and secondary infections, and how these classifications influence disease control strategies.
8. What is the role of molecular classification in the study of plant diseases? How has genetic analysis helped in categorizing plant diseases and understanding pathogen diversity?
9. Discuss the classification of plant diseases based on their mode of infection. Compare and contrast direct infection, systemic infection, and local infection in plants.
10. Explain the significance of integrated disease management in plant disease classification. How do various approaches (cultural, chemical, biological) help in managing diseases classified according to different factors?

7

Parasitism

Parasitism

The term parasitism refers to a parasite's taking of food from its host. Without chlorophyll, fungi are unable to synthesis their own sources of food. Fungi are classified into three main biological groups according on the basis of mode of the nutrient uptake . Parasites, Saprophytes and Symbionts, The term saprophytes, or saprobes, refers to those fungi that feed on dead and decaying organic matter (Gr. sapros rotten + bios life). Some of them have evolved farther, but they are still unable to grow on other living things and can only exist as saprobes. We refer to them as obligate saprophytes(L. Obligare = to bind sapros) . On the other hand, some species live as saprophytes, but under certain circumstances, they can infect another living entity. We refer to them as facultative parasites (Greek parasitos + Latin facultas ability). Many fungus infect living hosts and deprive them of their food. They are called parasites (Greek: parasitos, which means to eat beside). Additionally, a few of them developed into facultative soprophytes (L. facultatas ability + Gr. sapros) after diverging as obligatory parasites (L. Obligarę to bind + Gr. parasitos table mate). Obligate parasites can only grow in culture on living media; in the wild, they can only feed on living protoplasm. On the other hand, facultative saprophytes are basically parasitic organisms but also capable of growing on dead organic matter under some conditions.

Broad Categories of Parasitism

In fact, a number of fungi, once considered to be obligate parasites, have been cultured on artificial media. This makes the term obligate inappropriate Luttrell (1974) recognized three broad categories of parasitism which are as follows:

A. Biotrophs

These are those organisms which, regardless of the ease with which they can be cultured, in nature obtain their food from the living tissues on which they complete their life-cycles. Some typical examples are rusts, smuts and mildews

B. Hemibiotrophs

These are organisms which attack living tissues in the same way as biotrophs but continue to develop and sporulate after the tissue is dead. Typical examples of these are leaf-spotting fungi.

C. Necrotrophs

These are organisms which kill host tissues in advance of penetration and then live saprophytically. Sclerotium, Ventruria, Claviceps is the typical example.

Evolution of Parasitism

In contrast to their animal counterparts, plants attempt to coexist with their parasites by reducing the negative impacts of the latter. A parasite that is successful might also lessen the pressure on the plant at the same time. Because of these factors, symbiosis is regarded as the most developed type of parasitism. It seems sense to place saprotrophs at the bottom of the hypothetical parasitism hierarchy (Table-1)as they only inhabit dead organic material. Certain saprotrophs, such as Pythium sp., which possesses traits of a true saprophyte but is limited to attacking the tissues of young and succulent plants, have developed the ability to become parasites due to the fierce competition among them for the same source of organic matter. Due to their ability to target both more mature tissues and thinner tissues, pathogens like Rhizoctonia and Sclerotium can be regarded as more resilient. These pathogens have a broad range of hosts. They deploy chemical weapons, like as enzymes and secondary metabolites, to cause significant damage to the host tissues. They are necrotrophs. As one ascends the hypothetical parasitic hierarchy, necrotrophs emerge, exhibiting a greater reliance on their host and a reduced capacity for saprophytic survival. They rely more on toxins than on enzymes that break down walls. They result in significant tissue necrosis, although little to no tissue maceration occurs. More progress toward semibiotrophs and biotrophs has most likely been directed by:

1. Less reliance on enzymes and toxins by the pathogens.
2. Increased phytoharmone involvement.
3. A reduction in the parasites' harmful impact and a rise in their reliance on living host cells.
4. Reduced range of the host and
5. An increasing degree of synchronization between the parasite's and host's physiological processes.

Genetic synchronization-driven increases in physiological synchronization most likely contributed to the emergence of symbionts like mycorrhizae and lichens, where the parasite and host begin to benefit from one another. The host range of biotrophic symbionts is rather extensive, in contrast to that of biotrophic pathogens. This can be explained by three factors: (1) the parasite's capacity to get through the plant's general defenses; (2) the biotrophic relationship, which places less stress on the host plant; and (3) the advantages the host receives from its interaction with these biotrophs. If a pathogen can synchronize its physiological processes with the host's after it has penetrated the host's general defense barriers, it is considered to have achieved basic compatibility with the host. Merely establishing basic compatibility, however, does not ensure that, given the same environmental circumstances, every member of a specific host species would be equally susceptible to infection by all members of the pathogen.We refer to this second degree of host-parasite interaction as race-cultivar compatibility or specificity.

Table 1: Hypothetical hierarchical position of the different plant pathogens based on their parasitic advancement.

Degree of Synchronization		Fungi	Bacteria	Viruses/ Viroids	Nematodes	Mollecutes
	Symbiosis	Lichens, Vam Fungi	Rhizobium spp.			
	Biotrophs	Powdery Mildews Downy Mildews Rusts		Viroids Viruses	Secondary Endoparasites Migratory Endoparasites Ectoparasites	MLOs/ Spiro Plasma
	Semi-biotrophs	Phytophthora spp. Smuts	Agrobacterium spp.			
	Nectotrohs	Colletotrichum spp. Fusarium spp. Rhizoctonia spp.	Psudomonas spp. Xanthomonas spp. Clavibacter, RLB, Xylella, Sterptomyces			

Model Practice Question

A. Objective Questions

a. Multiple Choice Questions

1. Those organisms which requires living hosts or tissues complete their life cycle

   (a) Biotroph (b) Necrotroph

   (c) Hemibiotroph (d) All

2. These are organisms which kill host tissues in advance of penetration and then live saprophytically

   (a) Biotroph (b) Necrotroph

   (c) Hemibiotroph (d) All

3. These are organisms which attack living tissues in the same way as biotrophs but continue to develop and sporulate after the tissue is dead.

   (a) Biotroph (b) Necrotroph

   (c) Hemibiotroph (d) All

4. The organisms that are still unable to grow on other living things and can only exist as saprobes.

   (a) Obligate parasites (b) Facultative parasites

   (c) Obligate saprophyte (d) Facultative saprophyte

5. Those fungi that feed on dead and decaying organic matter are called

   (a) Saprophytes (b) Parasites

   (c) Symbionts (d) All

6. Those fungi that feed on living organisms are called

   (a) Saprophytes (b) Parasites

   (c) Symbionts (d) All

7. The host range of biotrophic symbionts is rather extensive, in contrast to that of biotrophic pathogens. This can be explained by which factors

   (1) The parasite's capacity to get through the plant's general defenses.

   (2) The blotrophic relationship, which places less stress on the host plant.

   (3) The advantages the host receives from its interaction with these biotrophs.

   (4) All

8. Rhizoctonia and Sclerotium is
   (a) Biotroph (b) Necrotroph
   (c) Hemibiotroph (d) All
9. Which one is an obligate parasite
   (a) Rusts (b) Smuts
   (c) Mildews (d) All
10. An organism that is ordinarily parasitic but under proper conditions may be saprophytic
   (a) Obligate parasites (b) Facultative parasites
   (c) Obligate saprophyte (d) Facultative saprophyte

Answer

Q. No.	Answer	Q. No	Answer
1	(a) Biotroph	6	(b) Parasites
2	(b) Necrotroph	7	(d) All
3	(c) Hemibiotroph	8	(b) Necrotroph
4	(c) Obligate saprophyte	9	(d) All
5	(a) Saprophytes	10	(d Facultative saprophyte

b. True/False

1. Fungi cannot synthesize their own food sources due to the presence of chlorophyll.
2. A number of fungi, once considered to be obligate parasites, have been cultured on artificial media.
3. Rust is a typical example of obligate parasite.
4. Unlike their animal counterparts, plants make an effort to live in harmony with their parasites by lessening the detrimental effects of the latter.
5. Powdey mildew is a typical example of facultative parasite.
6. The fungus Rhizoctonia is a typical example of necrotroph.
7. Symbiosis is regarded as the most developed type of parasitism.
8. Saprotrophs exist at the bottom of the hypothetical parasitism hierarchy as they only inhabit dead organic material.
9. Rhizoctonia and Sclerotium deploy chemical weapons, like as enzymes and secondary metabolites to cause significant damage to the host tissues.

10. Genetic synchronization-driven increases in physiological synchronization most likely contributed to the emergence of symbionts.

Answer

Q. No	Answer	Q. No	Answer
1	False	6	True
2	True	7	True
3	True	8	True
4	True	9	True
5	False	10	True

B. Descriptive Questions

a. Short answer questions

1. Differentiate between saprophyte and parasite with suitable examples.
2. Why symbiosis is regarded as the most developed type of parasitism.
3. Differentiate between obligate and facultative parasite.
4. Define Necrotroph.
5. Name three fungus having wide range of host.
6. Why sapostrophes exist at the bottom of the hypothetical parasitism hierarchy.
7. What is parasitism? Classify them in details with suitable examples.
8. Discuss in details about evolution of parasitism. Explain hypothetical hierarchical position of the different plant pathogens based on their parasitic advancement.

b. Long answer questions

1. Explain the concept of pathogenesis in plant pathology and how it relates to the interaction between a plant and a pathogen.
2. Describe the different stages of pathogenesis in plant diseases, from pathogen entry to disease development, and explain the key events that occur at each stage.
3. Discuss the role of virulence factors in the pathogenesis of plant diseases. How do virulence factors contribute to the ability of pathogens to infect and damage plants?
4. What are the different types of plant pathogens (fungi, bacteria, viruses, nematodes, etc.), and how does their mechanism of infection and pathogenesis differ?

5. Examine the role of plant defense mechanisms in combating pathogen invasion. How do plants recognize and respond to pathogens at the molecular level during the process of pathogenesis?
6. What is the role of plant hormones, such as jasmonic acid, salicylic acid, and ethylene, in regulating the plant's response to pathogen infection? Discuss their involvement in the pathogenesis process.
7. How do environmental factors, such as temperature, humidity, and soil conditions, influence the pathogenesis of plant diseases? Provide examples of how different environmental conditions can either exacerbate or mitigate disease progression.
8. Explain the process of pathogen evolution and how it affects the pathogenesis of plant diseases. How do pathogens adapt to overcome plant defenses over time?
9. Discuss the concept of host specificity in plant pathogens. How does the genetic makeup of both the plant and the pathogen determine the outcome of an infection?
10. Describe the various methods used to study the pathogenesis of plant diseases in the laboratory. How do these methods help researchers understand the mechanisms behind infection and develop strategies for disease control?

8

Development of Disease in Plants (Pathogenesis)

Most often, a plant gets diseased when it is harmed by an abiotic agents or attacked by a pathogen. As a result, in the first scenario, interaction and contact between the pathogen and the plant are required for the occurrence of a plant disease. No disease develops even though a pathogen and a plant come into contact if the weather is too extreme at the time of the pathogen's contact with the plant and for a while afterwards. This could be because the plant is able to fend off the pathogen's attack or because the pathogen is unable to attack at all. Therefore, it would appear that in order for disease to manifest, a third component—a set of environmental factors falling within a favorable range—must also exist. The degree of disease severity in both individual plants and plant populations is impacted by changes in any one of the three components, which can each show significant fluctuation. Plants can exhibit genetic uniformity over a wide area, be of a species or variety that may be more or less resistant to the pathogen, or they may be too young or too old for the pathogen to prefer. All of these factors can either accelerate or slow down the rate at which a particular pathogen causes disease. The way the three elements of disease interact has frequently been represented as a triangle (Fig. 2-1), which is commonly known as the "disease triangle." Every angle of the triangle symbolizes one of the three elements. The totality of each component's attributes that promote disease determines the length of each side. If the plants are susceptible, at a susceptible stage of growth, or densely planted, the host side would be long and the potential amount of disease could be large. In contrast, if the plants are resistant, the wrong age, or widely spaced, the host side — and the amount of disease — would be small or zero. The larger the potential amount of disease, the longer the pathogen side would be. Furthermore, the longer the environment side would be and the higher the potential amount of disease, the more favorable environmental circumstances would be that support the pathogen (such as temperature, moisture, and wind) or that lower host resistance. The area of the triangle would represent the quantity of disease in a plant or in a plant population if the three elements of the disease triangle could be quantified. Should any one of the three elements be zero, there may be no disease. The terms for the three components of the disease—host plant, pathogen, and environment—are alternatively shown as a triangle with the triangle's peaks instead of its sides.

Stages in the development of disease: The disease cycle

A sequence of relatively unique events leads to the establishment and perpetuation of the pathogen and the disease in every infectious disease. We refer to this chain of events as a disease cycle or pathogenesis. A disease cycle can occasionally resemble the life cycle of the pathogen pretty closely, but it mostly relates to how the pathogen causes the disease to manifest, progress, and persist rather than the pathogen itself. The disease cycle covers periods within a growing season and from one growing season to the next and encompasses changes in the plant and its symptoms as well as those in the pathogen. The primary events in a disease cycle are

1. Inoculation

Inoculation is the coming in contact of a pathogen with a plant. Inoculum defined as the part of the pathogen, which on contact with a suitable host cause infection. E.g. of fungal inoculum; chlaymydospores, sclerotia, oospores teleutospores, zoospores, conidiospores etc. In bacteria, mollicutes, the inoculum is whole individual. One to the unit of inoculum of the adult nematodes, nematode juveniles, pathogen is called propagule.

(a) Types of Inoculum

All inoculum that survives in the winter or summer and causes the infection in the spring or autumn is called primary inoculum, and the it causes are called primary infections. An inoculum produced from primary infections is called secondary inoculum and it in turn causes secondary infections.

b) Source of Inoculums

- Sowing and planting materials *viz*., seeds, tubers, bulbs, rhizomes.
- Diseased plants in the field.
- Debris left on the land or used in compost heaps.
- Host plants in a dormant stage when conditions are not favorable.
- Soil infected with certain soil borne pathogens.

Plant diseases are spread in various ways:

1. Spread through seeds and other planting materials such as tubers, corm etc.
2. Spread by natural agents such as wind, water and rain.
3. Spread by animal and insects.

2. Penetration

The penetration process has two phases:

i) Pre penetration stage

During the pre penetration stage the fungus hyphae attach with the host surface. The spores will germinate or spores to produce germ tube or infection threads. This stage may be abortive if environments do not favor growth of the hypha or germination of spores.

ii) Penetration

During penetration, the infection thread enters the host by any of the following methods

(a) Entry through natural openings like stomata & lenticels.

b) Entry through rupture of the host surface due to development of organs like prop roots.

c) Entry through wounds due to mechanical injury or insect injury.

d) Direct penetration

The pathogen exerts its own effort to break the host barrier and directly enter through cuticle or epidermis without seeking the wounds or natural opcnings. Host barriers can be either structural barriers or chemical barriers. Enzymes produced by the pathogen will break down the epidermal cells and thus gain entry. Pathogens penetrate plant surfaces by direct penetration. Some fungi penetrate tissues in one way only, others bacteria enter plant mostly through wounds, less frequently through natural opening and never directly. Viruces, viroids, mollicutes and protozoa enter through wound made by vectors, although some viruses and viroids may also enter through wounds made by tools and other means. Nematodes enter plants by direct penetration and sometimes through natural openings. Penetration does not always lead to infection.

3. Infection

Infection is the process by which pathogen establish contact with the susceptible cells or tissues of the host and take nutrient from them. During infection pathogens grow or multiply or both within the plant tissues and invade and colonize the plant to a lesser or greater extent. Therefore, invasion of the plant tissues by the pathogen and growth and reproduction of the pathogen (colonization) in or on infected tissues are actual two concurrent sub stages of disease development within the stage of infection. Successful infections result in the appearance of symptom on the host plant. In most plant diseases, symptoms appear from a few days to few weeks after inoculation.

4. Colonization

Various pathogen invade hosts in different ways and to different extents. Mon fungi spread into all the tissues of the plant organs they infect, either by grown directly through the cells as an intracellular mycelium or by growing between the cells as an intercellular mycelium. The fungi that cause vascular wilts invad the xylem vessels of plants. Bacteria invade tissues intercellularly, although where part of the cell wall dissolve, bacteria also grow intracellular. Bacteria causing vascular wilt, invade the xylem vessels. Viruses, viroids, mollicutes, fastidiou bacteria and protozoa invade tissues by moving from cell to cell intercelluarly. Viruses and viroids invade all types of living plant cells, mollicutes and protozoa invade phloem sieve tubes and perhaps a few adjacent phloem parenchymatous cells. Most nematodes invade tissues intercellularly, but some can invade intracellularly-many nematodes do not invade cells or tissues at all but feed by piercing epidermal cells with their styles.

5. Growth and Reproduction of the Pathogen

Individual fungi and parasitic higher plants generally invade and infect tissues by growing into them from one initial point of inoculation. Most of these pathogens, whether producing a small spot, a large infected area, or a general necrosis of the plant continue to grow and branch out within the infected host indefinitely so that the same pathogen individual spread into more and more plant tissues until the spread at the infection is stopped or the plant is dead. All other pathogens like bacteria, virus, viroids, nematodes and protozoa, do not increase much, at all, in size with time, since, their size and shape remain relatively unchanged throghout their existance. These pathogens invade and infect new tissues within the plant by reproducing at a rapid rate and increasing their number tremendous in the infected tissues. The progeny may then be carried passively through:

(a) Plasmadesmata: virus and viroids

b) Phloem: viruses, viroids, mollicutes protozoa, some fastidious bacteria

c) Xylem: some bacteria, nematodes

6. Dissemination of the Pathogen

Following the infection, the pathogen will continue its growth, produce spores or reproductive units, which will find exit through host surface and spread to repeat the same process. Many pathogens spread through crops in a special and often spectacular way. Some cover tremendous distances at a remarkable speed, especially pathogens with airborne propagules, like rusts. Pathogens which infect subterranean plant organs exhibit a restricted pattern of dispersal. Then there are pathogens which depend for their dispersal of spores and propagules on rain or water, while others need a vector like man, insects and nematodes. Some parasites are transported with seed, thus depending on the hosts own dispersal processes.

There are many dispersal mechanisms. Some of these mechanisms are both elegant and highly efficient in that they are closely adapted to the biology of the host, like the synchronization of spore release in certain pathogens like Venturia and Claviceps. Other parasites produce millions of spores, saturating the environment with propagules in an apparently haphazard and wasteful way.

7. Survival of Pathogen

Pathogens must find some alternate source of their survival in the absence of their cultivated host; otherwise the infection chain will be remaining incomplete. Infection chain is the chain of events leading to the completion of pathogenesis.

The source of survival can be grouped into

(a) Infected host as reservoir of inoculums

  i. Cultivated host: Main host

  ii. Collateral host: Wild host of the same family

  iii. Alternate host: Wild host of other family

b) Saprophytic survival outside the host. Soil and plant debris serve as the media for survival. E.g. Pythium, Rhizoctonia

c) Dormant organs of pathogen as a source of survival and primary inoculums; only fungi and nematodes have spores and cysts etc, while virus and bacteria have no resting stage.

The Disease Triangle and Disease Pyramid

The disease triangle is one of the first concepts encountered by students in an introductory plant pathology course and often may be encountered in higher level classes. The interactions of the three component namely *(1) susceptible host (2) virulent pathogen* and *(3) favorable environments* have been visualized as a triangle, generally referred to as the "*Disease Traingle*". Some plant pathologists have elaborated on the Disease Triangle by adding one or more parameters. Suggested additional parameters may be *human activity, vectors* and *time.* A three dimensional disease triangle may result in four dimensional *Disease Pyramid* or *Disease Tetrahedron* after addition of a single parameter.

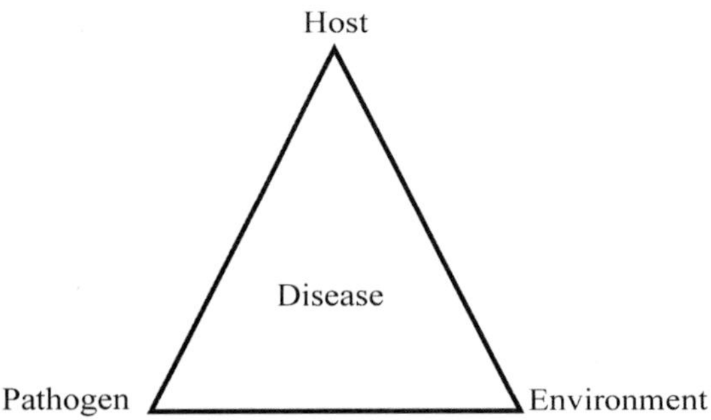

Development of epidemic requires interaction of a highly virulent pathogen and a susceptible host in an environment that favours the development of disease. The environment can affect both the susceptibility of host and the activity of the pathogen . The pathogen can affect the host and the host can influence the environment. An understanding of these factors and their interactions for a particular disease in a particular locality allows prediction of disease outbreaks and intervention to reduce the amount of disease.

Factors Affecting Disease Development

There are three major factors that affect disease development

1. Pathogen factors
2. Host factors
3. Environmental factors

   1. Pathogen factors
      - Presence of pathogen
      - Pathogenicity (virulence and aggressiveness)
      - Adaptability
      - Dispersal efficiency
      - Survival efficiency
      - Reproductive fitness
   2. Host factors
      - Susceptibility
      - Growth stage and form
      - Population density and structure
      - General health

3. Environmental factors
    - Temperature
    - Rainfall
    - Dew
    - Leaf wetness period
    - Soil temperature
    - Soil moisture
    - Soil fertility
    - Air pollution

1. Pathogen factors

(a) **Presence of pathogen:** The main factor which determines whether or no disease occurs at all is the presence or absence of the pathogen. In the out break of late blight of potato in north India, the presence of absence of the pathogen is the overriding factor that determines whether or not disease occurs.

b) **Pathogenicty:** The amount of disease that develops if often determined by pathogenicity of the prevalent population of the pathogen. The term pathogenicity comprises both the virulence of the pathogen and its aggresivenenss .It also includes aspects of dispersal and survival fitness. Control of diseases often involves monitoring the pathogenicity of the prevailing pathogen population as a guide to the breeding of resistant crop varieties.

c) **Adaptibility:** The adaptability of pathogen is very important in determining its ability to overcome resistance in newly released varieties or to adapt to the changed environmental conditions. It is governed by the genetic flexibility of the pathogen population and its reproductive efficiency. *Puccinia graminis* has high reproductive efficiency and so is likely to adapt very fast where as *O. theobromae* on cocoa has a much lower reproductive capacity and so likely to adapt more slowly.

d) **Dispersal efficiency:** The ability of a pathogen to cause destructive disease epidemics depends on its ability to disperse rapidly over long distances. The urediniospores of rust can be blown long distances in a few days , allowing epidemics to develop rapidly over very large areas. Soil borne pathogens, on the other hand, have limited dispersal ability and tends to cause localized disease outbreaks.

e) **Survival efficiency:** The ability of a pathogen to cause disease in successive seasons depends on its ability to survive. *Plasmodiophora brassicae*, the cause of club roots of crucifers, form spores that enable the pathogens to survive in the soil for many years, thus reducing the effectiveness of disease control using crop rotation. The sclerotia of *Sclerotium rolfsii* and Sclerotinia spp. are also particularly effective in enabling these pathogens to survive through the summer and winter, resulting in larger quantities of inoculums to initiate epidemics in the new growing season.

2. Host factors

(a) **Susceptibility:** The occurrence of individuals in the host population that are *susceptible* to the particular pathogen is the main factor affecting disease development. For a disease epidemic to occur, the host plant population must be largely susceptible to attack by the pathotypes of the pathogen in the vicinity. The most important means of disease management is to plant varieties that are not susceptible to the prevailing population of the pathogen of concern.

b) **Growth stage and form:** The growth stage and form of the host greatly influence the occurrence of disease. The growth stage also determines the degree of closure of the canopy, which in turn affect the microclimate within the canopy. Some diseases such as damping off are more common in seedlings, while others are characteristic of mature plants.

c) **Population density and structure:** The characteristics of population structure and density in the host will have a large bearing on the development of disease in the population. Many plant diseases are much more common in dense than in sparse plantings. Modern intensive agriculture provide and ideal situation for development of plant disease because variety or even clones derived from a single plant are commonly planted over a large area with few or no individuals of non host species or cultivars interfere with inoculums dispersal. Spectecular disease epidemics have occurred when susceptible host varieties were planted over large areas or when a new pathogen was introduced such plantations. Such a situation occurred with the spread of late blight of potato to Ireland in the 1840s and with the spread of coffee rust to Ceylon in the 1870s. Both pathogens encountered extensive monocultures of their respective hosts, potato and coffee and caused destructive epidemics.

d) **General health:** The prior health of the host is often important in determining the occurrence of disease. Necrotrophic pathogens are often more damaging on poorly growing than on vigorous hosts while opposite is the cause of biotrophs.

3. Environmental factors

The total environment encompasses the whole biosphere within which the epidemiologic processes join up. The total environment is divided into micro, meso and macro-environemnt for easy understanding.

The *microenvironment* is the space in which the epidemiologic processes at cell and organ level occur. The largest part of the infection cycle, from *deposition to takeoff*. The microenvironment of the leaves is called phyllosphere, which includes a laminar air layer of up to 1mm in thickness surrounding the leaf. The *phyllosphere* is a *three dimensional space*, whereas the actual leaf surface, or *phylloplane*, is a *two dimensional space*. In regard to the roots there is a three dimensional rhizosphere (Hiltner, 1904) and a two dimensional *rhizoplane.*

The mesoenvironment is formed by the crop.It is formed by the plants and simultaneously it influences the plants and the epidemiologic processes in the crop.

The macroenvironment is the air layer from the crop surface to the trophosphere. Some epidemiologic processes of extreme importance occur in the macroenvironment. There are three major environemental factors that affect disease development are

(a) **Tempcrature:** Temperature affects *Latent period*: the time between infection and the first appearance of disease symptoms, *Generation time*: the time between infection and sporulation and *Infectious period*: the time during which the pathogen continues producing propagules. At higher temperatures the disease cycle is speed up with the result that epidemics develop faster. Under cooler conditions, epidemics progress is usually slower. So disease incidence and severity may not reach the threshold level necessary to cause significant crop loss.

b) **Moisture:** Moisture is the most important environmental factor influencing disease outbreak caused by fungi, bacteria and nematode. The term "moisture" cover *rainfall, relative humidity, dew* and *leaf wetness.* The influence of rain splash and running water on dispersal of pathogen propagules is also important. Leaf wetness is a more accurate predictor of disease than rainfall and dew period. We often the combination of leaf wetness and ambient temperature is critical in determining the proporation of pathogen propagules that infect the host. Moisture has an important effect on dispersal of pathogens. Free water or the impact of raindrops facilitates the liberation and dispersal of many fungi and nearly all bacteria. This is very useful adaptation for a pathogen because when the propagules are dispersed, conditions are also likely to be suitable for germination and infection. For examples coelomycetes produce wet spores that are picked up by rain splash and dispersed. Many dry spores are liberated by the force of impact of raindrops.

Soil borne diseases are affected mainly by the environmental conditions in the soil. Wetness is often a critical factor. Some pathogens like pythiaceous fungi causing damping off require a period of soil saturation to allow germination of survival prpagules and infection of roots. The zoospores of pythecious fungi require free water for their release and mobility.

c) **Soil fertility :** Soil fertility can affect development of both soil and soil borne disease. Some facultative pathogens cause more disease when plants are growing poorly under conditions of nutrient deficiency. On the other hand biotrophic pathogens such as rusts and powdery mildews are often more common on vigorous well fertilized plants than on poorly growing plants.

The organic matter content of soil has an important influence on some soil borne pathogens. For example, eucalyptus dieback is common in sandy or gravelly soils low in organic matter. Successful management of *P. cinnamomi* in avocado has been achieved by greatly increasing the organic matter content. Soils high in organic matter contain larger populations of antagonistic microorganisms which reduce the survival time of plant pathogens and the subsequent incidence of disease.

d) **Pollution:** The aerial environment has been observed to affect plant disease. In regions where aerial pollution associated with industrial development has been especially great, the concentration of pollutant like oxide of sulphur and nitrogen can affect disease development and in the form of acid rain, can directly damage plants.

Model Practice Questions

A.Objective Type Questions

a. Multiple Choice Questions

1. The interactions of the three components of disease have often been visualized as a triangle generally referred to as the

(a) Disease Triangle (b) Disease Pyramid

(c) Disease Hierarchy (d) All

2. This chain of events leading to the development of the disease is called a

(a) Pathogenesis (b) Pathogenicity

(c) Virulence (d) Aggressiveness

3. The initial contact of a pathogen with a site of plant where infection is possible
   (a) Inoculation (b) Penetration
   (c) Infection (d) Colonization
4. The entry of pathogen inside the host is called
   (a) Inoculation (b) Penetration
   (c) Establishment of infection (d) Colonization
5. The establishment of host parasitic relationships is called
   (a) Inoculation (b) Penetration
   (c) Infection (d) Colonization
6. Plant diseases are spread in various ways:
   (a) Spread through seeds and other planting materials
   b) Spread by natural agents such as wind, water and rain.
   c) Spread by animal and insects.
   d) All
7. The time between infection and the first appearance of disease symptoms,
   (a) Latent period (b) Generation time
   (c) Infectious period (d) Time period
8. The time between infection and sporulation
   (a) Latent period (b) Generation time
   (c) Infectious period (d) Time period
9. The time during which the pathogen continues producing propagules
   (a) Latent period (b) Generation time
   (c) Infectious period (d) Time period
10. Which plant pathogens produce systemic infections?
   (a) Mollicutes (b) Viroids
   (c) Viruses (d) All

Answer

Q. No	Answer	Q. No	Answer
1	(a) Disease Triangle	6	(d) All
2	(a) Pathogenesis	7	(a) Latent period
3	(a) Inoculation	8	(b) Generation time
4	(b) Penetration	9	(c) Infectious period
5	(c) Infection	10	(d) All

b. True/False

1. Disease develops when a pathogen and a plant come into contact.
2. The length of each side is proportional to the sum total of the characteristics of each component that favor disease.
3. There cannot be a disease if any one of the three factors like host, pathogen and environment is zero.
4. There may be multiple infection cycles inside one disease cycle in some diseases.
5. Pathogenicity comprises both the virulence of the pathogen and its aggresivenenss.
6. Penetration does not always lead to infection.
7. Viruses and viroids invade all types of living plant cells.
8. Leafhoppers are the main vectors of mollicutes, fastidious bacteria, and protozoa.
9. Soil inhabitants are able to survive indefinitely as saprophytes.
10. Bacteria, nematodes, and spores and mycelial fragments of fungi present in the soil are disseminated by rain or irrigation water.

Answer

Q. No	Answer	Q. No	Answer
1	True	6	True
2	True	7	True
3	True	8	True
4	True	9	True
5	False	10	True

B. Descriptive Question

a. Short answers

1. Which of the following two statements are correct and why?
   a. Disease cycle is an alternate name of the life cycle of a pathogen.
   b. Disease cycle represents the life cycle of the disease, not the life cycle of the pathogen that causes the disease.
2. How root-cap border cells are related to the infection in soil-borne diseases?
3. Name any two attractants stimulants of soil-borne pathogens.
4. Which bacterial pathogen is called ‘natural genetic engineer’ and why?

5. What is 'infection cushion'?
6. Which category of pathogens develop haustoria? Mention possible functions of haustoria apart from nutrient uptake.

b. Long answers

1. Explain the following: i. Infection ii. Latent infection iii. Invasion iv. Colonization v. Inoculum potential
2. Describe the general principles of plant infection? How infection is caused in some of the important plant pathogen fungi and bacteria.
3. What is infection? Describe in detail the mechanism of infection and establishment of any typical fungal pathogen.
4. What are the different stages in the development of a infectious plant disease. Describe in detail the pre penetration activities of fungal pathogens. Gives suitable examples.
5. Describe various aspects of a typical disease-cycle.
6. Discuss in detail the prepenetration phase of infection.
7. Write notes on:
   a. Chemotaxis
   b. Melanized appressoria
   c. Pathogen adhesion on host
   d. Infection plaques
8. Discuss the growth of pathogen superficially, subcuticularly, and endophytically in their hosts.

9

Fungi and Their Morphology, Reproduction and Classification of Fungi

Definition

Fungi are eukaryotic, spore bearing, *achlorophyllus, heterotrophic* and thallophytic plants with varied forms and habitats, representing heterothallic or homothallic types of sexuality with characteristic sexual and /or asexual means of reproduction without tissue differentiation.

General Characteristics of Fungi

1. Thallus

The body of the fungus is called as **Thallus**, which is without stem, root and leaves. It may be Plasmodial, Pseudoplasmodial , Pseudomycelial or Mycelial. A single thread like filament is called as **hypha.** A hypha is made up of a thin, transparent tabular wall filled or lined with a layer of protoplasm.

A group of hypha constituting the body of fungus is called as **mycelium** may be septate or aseptate. i.e **coenocytic**.

(a) **Coenocytic or Nonseptate or Aseptate Mycelium:** When mycelium is not divided by cross walls called as **Coenocytic** mycelium. Depending upon the nature of parasitism with the host plant, mycelium is either ecotophytic or endophytic.

b) **Septate Mycelium:** When mycelium is divided by cross walls or septa called as **septate** mycelium.

i) **Ecotophytic Mycelium:** The hyphae grows on external/epidermal surface by means of special sucking organs called as **haustoria.** is called **ecotophytic mycelium** e.g. Powdery Mildew Fungi.

ii) **Endophytic Mycelium:** When hyphae grows inside the epidermal layer of plant or host tissues, is called as **endophytic mycelium**. e.g. Aspergilus fungi. Endophytic mycelium is of following types.

(a) Intercellular
(b) Intracellular
(c) Vascular

(a) Intercellular Mycelium: Mycelium growing in between the cells.

b) Intracellular Mycelium: Mycelium growing within the host cell. e. g Smut fungi.

c) Vascular Mycelium: Mycelium growing in vascular tissues of the plant. e. g Wilts

2. Cell Wall

Cell wall is well defined, typically chitinised which contains **chitin or cellulose** or both (Cellulose in oomycetes), living structure of the cell called as organelles (Cytoplasm, nucleolus and protoplasm). Nonliving structure of the cell called as Inorganelles (Chitin , cellulose).

3. Nutrition

Nutrition is **heterotrophic** i.e. Photosynthesis lacking and absorptive (They lack chlorophyll and can't manufacture their own food from CO2 and water). Their mechanism of nourishment is **absorption** which takes place by **osmosis** through the cell walls.

Fungi are divided into three groups according to the manner they obtain their food as:

a. Saprophytes

Those organism which requires dead organic matter to complete its life cycle as saprophytes. e.g. Mucor and Rhizophus.

b. Symbionts or Symbiosis

When two dissimilar organisms lives together in close association for mutual benefits is called as **symbiosis**. When two or more organisms lives together in close association for mutual benefits is called as **mutualism**.e.g. Lichen- Fungus and algae Mycorrhiza- Fungi and roots of higher forest plants.

c. Parasites

An organism that lives within or upon another living organism from which it derives nourishment and in which it may cause various degrees of injury is called as **parasite** or An organism which completely depends on its host for food called as **parasite.**

Among the parasite one can distinguish different degree of parasitism as i) Obligate parasites ii) Non obligate parasites, iii) Facultative saprophytes iv) Facultative parasites.

i) Obligate Parasites or Biotrophs

Those organisms which requires living hosts or tissues complete their life cycle , are called as obligate parasites or An obligate parasite is an organism that can live only on living tissue. They can never be grown on dead, artificial food material. Rust, mildews, viruses.

ii) Non Obligate Parasites or Necrotrophs

Those organisms when kills the tissue in advance of penetration and then lives on it as saprophytically. E.g. *Sclerotium, Ventruria, Claviceps,*

iii) Facultative Saprophytes

An organism that is ordinarily parasitic but under proper conditions may be saprophytic. e.g. *Smut, Sphacelotheca* sp.

iv) Facultative Parasites

An organism that is ordinarily saprophytic but under proper conditions may be parasitic. e.g. *Pythium, Phytophthora.*

4. Nuclear Status

Fungi multinucleate, mycelium being homocakaryotic or heterokaryotic or haploid or diploid or dikarytoic limited duration. Well defined structures i.e. nuclear membrane, nucleolus, and chromatin material etc.

5. Sexuality

Asexual, Sexual or and homo or heterothallic.

6. Life Cycle

Simple to Complex.

7. Sporocarps

Microscopic or macroscopic and showing limited differentiation.

8. Distribution

Cosmopolitan.

Definition of Fungus and Somatic Structures

Definition

Fungus is Latin word meaning **'mushroom'**

Alexopoulus and Mims 1979 defined fungus as eukaryotic or nucleated spore bearing , achlorophyllous organism generally produced by sexual or asexual method and whose filamentous branched somatic structure is typically covered by cell wall and cell wall further consists of either cellulose or chitin or glucon or some other complex organic carbohydrate.

Somatic Structures

1. Haustoria

A modified mycelial branch that grows into a plant cell, makes intimate contact with the protoplast, and absorbs food. They are of different shapes and size ranging from knob like structures to simple, lobed, branched, and coiled and they are able to penetrate only in the cell wall and not in the plasma membrane.

2. Appressoria

These are localized swellings of the tip of germ tube or older hyphae that develop in response to contact with the host. In simple these are special structures for attachment in the early stage of infection. Form these a minute infection peg usually grows and enters the **epidermal** cell of the host.

Types of Fungal Thalli

1. Homothallic Fungi: Gr. *homo*= same + *thallos* = shoot, tallus): Fungi in which sexual reproduction takes place in a single thallus or If male and f male sex organs or both the gametes are produced on the same thallus, they are self fertile or self compatible. e.g. Powdery mildew of mung –*Sapharotheca fulginae.*

2. Hetrothallic Fungi: -(Gr. *Hetero*= different + *thallos* = shoot, tallus). If male and female sex organs or both the gametes are produced on the different thallus, they are self sterile or self incompatible. e.g. Rust Fungi.

Fungus Tissue

1. Plectenchyma; During certain stages of fungal development, the mycelium becomes organized into loosely or compact woven tissues, as against the loose hyphae ordinarily found in the mycelium. The organized fungal tissues are called **Plectenchyma.**

The Plectenchyma is of two Types

a. **Prosenchyma:** The loosely woven tissue in which the component hyphae with elongated cells lie more or less parallel to one another is called prosenchyma.

b. **Pseudoparenchyma:** The fungal tissues which ar closely packed, in the form of more or less isodiametric or oval cells resembling the parenchyma cells of higher plants are called pseudoparenchyma. Both prosenchyma and pseudoparenchyma compose various type of vegetative and reproductive structures. Both stromata and sclerotia are somatic structure of fungi.

Modification of Mycelium or Thallus

Rhizomorphs

The mycelium of some fungi forms thick strands, in such strands the hyphae lose their individuality and form complex tissues. The strand are called rhizomorph (root like structures). Its function is believed to be the transportation of water across dry areas. The cables are usually large enough to be readily viewed without a microscope and resemble small roots of a seed plant. They belongs to subdivision basidiomycotina. e.g. *Arnillaria millea*

Stroma or Stromata

It is a compact mass of the hyphae and appears as pseudoparenchymatous tissue and contain fruiting body of the fungus. e.g. ergot of bajara.

Sclerotium

Asexual, thickwalled, multicelled, overseasoning structure. Masses of cells that form a hard, rounded structure with a differentiated rind in or a host. It may remain dormant for long periods and germinate under favourable conditions. e.g. *Sclerotium* spp.

Dormant Mycelium

It is the mycelium which hibernates in the host tissue to tide over unfavourable conditions, if remains in a dormant condition for a part of its life cycle and come up into activity when conditions are favourable. e.g. Loose smut of wheat, Downey mildew of grape, Koleroga of arecanut.

Gemmae

These are the chamydospores produced in lower fungi whose walls are thinner. They occur either singly or in chains a becomes separated after maturing. Gemmae break free from the mycelium and disperse in water. e.g. Mucor sp, Saprolegnia sp.

Spores in Fungi

The fungi reproduce by spores. Spores is a minute reproductive or propagative bodies functioning as a seed of fungi. These are produced in three ways.

1. Vegetatively
2. Asexually
3. Sexually

Spores:

There are three types of spores:

1) Vegetative

i) Chlamydospores

2) Asexual

i) Exogenous .e.g. Conidia, Oidia

ii) Endogenous: a. Non motile e.g. Aplanospores, b. Motile, e.g. Zoospores,

3) Sexual

i) Zygote

ii) Zygospores

iii) Oospores

iv) Ascospores

v) Basidiospores

I) Vegetative Spores in Fungi

Chlamydospores

A thick-walled asexual resting spore formed by the modification of a fungus hypha. They may be formed terminally or intercalary.e.g. *Fusarium* spp.

II) Asexual Spores in Fungi

Asexual spores form without nuclear fusion or act of breeding. These spores borne of sporophores. They are not usually resistance to unfavourable conditions. They are capable of rapid multiplication. They may be one or many celled borne on specialized hyphae or produced in special structures called as spores fruits.

a. Endogenous: (Produced inside)

These spores are formed internally within swollen sac by the division of protoplasm. e.g. Sporangiospores.

i) Sporangiospores

Sporangiospores are produced in a sac or sporangium and are hyaline, unicellular. These spores are liberated by breaking the wall of sporangium. When sporangium gives motile spores, it is known as zoosporangium and the spores as **zoospores.** These spores are **motile** by means of **flagella.**

ii) Aplanospore

A non motile spore produced in the sporangium is knows as **Aplanospore.**

b. Exogenous: (Produced outside)

These spores are borne externally on sporophores. e. g. Conidia, Oidia.

i) Conidia

These spores are produced on sepecialized hyphae i.e. conidiphore. Conidia differ in their size, shape, septation, colour, and branching within the same species.Conidia may be uni or multicellular, hyaline or coloured. e.g. *Alternaria, Helminthosporium.*

ii) Oidia

These spores are barrel shaped or rectangular in shape and are produced asexually in chains on the stalk called as oidiophore. e.g. Oidia in powdery mildew.

III) Sexual Spores in Fungi

The sexual spores are formed by the fusion between two gametes of opposite sec. Cell carrying the gamete is called gametangium and gamete is unisexual or haploid.

i) Oospores

It is the result of union between female gametes i.e. Oogonium and male gametes i.e. Antheridium. Anthridial nuclei passes to Oogonium through fertilization tube. The Oospores are thick walled and may be smooth or rough, dark in colour. These spores can resist the adverse conditions. e.g. Fungi of sub-division Mastigomycotian.

ii) Zygospores

A fungal resting spore produced by the fusion of equal gametes designated as +ve and –ve. The resultant spore is thick walled or spiny. The wall consists of two layer. Outer one is known as exosporium and inner layer as endosporium. These spores resist unfavourable conditions and germinate during favourable season. e.g. Fungi of sub-division zygomycotina.

iii) Zygote

It is form by union of to opposite haploid motile gametes. e.g. Lower fungi of the subdivision Mastigomycotiana.

iv) Ascospores

Ascospores is a result of union between male gamete. i.e. Antheridium and female gametes. i.e. Ascogonium. Anthridial nuclei passes to Oogonium through trichogyne. Ascospores are produce in a sanction as ascus and are generally eight in number. Ascospores may be single or many celled, hyaline or coloured and having various shapes. e.g. Fungi of sub-division Ascomycotina.

v) Basidiospores

A haploid spore formed externally on a basidium on a short stalk or tube known as sterigmata. They are produced exogenously and usually four in number. In these fungi sex organs are absent, except in rust fungi. e.g. Fungi of sub-division Basidiomycotina.

Spore Fruit in Fungi

A spore fruit is an aggregation of spores and spores bearing hyphae, sometimes naked but frequent enclosed in various types of containers or spore cases or receptacles. The spores fruit have a thick wall known as peridium.

Importance Spore Fruit in fungi

- The spore fruits are vital in tiding over unfavourable conditions, multiplication and maintenance of inoculum.
- The spore fruit are utilized as taxonomic characters in determining the broad lines of various groups of fungi.

Spore Fruit

There are two types of spores fruit based on whether spore fruit contains the sexual spore or asexual spores.

i) Asexual

a. Sporangium

b. Sorus

c. Coremium

d. Sporodochium

e. Pycnidium

f. Aecium

g. Acervulus

h. Pycnium

ii) Sexual

a. Ascocarps e.g. Cleistothecium, Apothecium, Perithecium

b. Basidiocarps e.g. Puffballs, Todstool

Asexual Spore Fruits in Fungi

1. Sporangium

This type of spore fruit is a characteristic of the fungi belonging to sub division mastigomycotina and zygomycotina. The elliptical sporangia are formed by the lower fungi belonging to subdivision mastigomycotina, which are semi-acquatic in nature, while round sporangia are formed by terrestrial fungi belonging to sub division zygomycotina

2. Aecium

Aecium is a inverted cup like or bell shaped structure usually formed on lower surface of the leaf, consisting of binuclear hyphal cells producing yellow or orange coloured spores which are usually formed in basipetal manner called **aeciosopores.**

3. Pycnium

A flask shaped structure containing Pycniospores and spermatia. e.g. Rust fungi.

4. Acervulus

It is compact mass of hyphae giving rise to short, simple hyaline condiophores, closely packed together forming cushion like mass with or without setae. It is also known as modified open sorus. e.g. *Collectrotrichum* and *Gleosporium.*

5. Pycnidium

Asexual, closed, ostiolate fruiting body with short conidiophores lining inner side which bear spores or conidia called Pycnidiospores. The spore fruit usually have an opening is called ostiole. e.g. *Phoma* sp. and *Phomopsis* sp.

6. Sporodochium

A spore fruit having cushion shaped Stroma, covered with conidiophores is known as **sporodochium.** The conidia formed inside and ooze out in sticky mass. e.g. Genus *Nectria, Fusarium.*

7. Synnemata

The hyphae, which form conidiophores and erect condiophores, grouped together to form **coremia**. Each Coremium consists of sterile stalk terminating into fertile hyphae bearing conidia. e. g. *Stysannus thyroseides*.

8. Sorus

It is little heap like compact mass of sporophores and spore which usually are covered by epidermis. At maturity, the epidermis breaks and the spores get liberated. e.g. Smut and rust.

Sexual Spore Fruit in Fungi

Ascocarps

Ascocarp is the spore fruit produced by the fungi belonging to the sub-division ascomycotina Sexual spore produced endogenously are known as **Ascospores** in sac like structure called **ascus**. The spore fruit are of various forms viz. Spherical shaped, flask, cup, saucer and pod shaped etc.

Following are the different types of Ascocarps

1. Apothecium

An open, cuplike, or saucer-shaped sexual fungal fruiting body containing asci.. The asci are arranged in palisade layer called hymenium. e.g. *Sclerotinia.*

2. Perithecium

A flask shaped ascocarp with narrow neck like having ostiole through which asci are released. The asci are arranged or lined the inner wall of the perithecium. The sterile structures present in between the asci known as paraphyses which help asci in nutrition and dispersion. e.g. *Claviceps* and *Glomerella.*

3. Cleistothecium

It is closed, sexual fruiting body of the ascomycetes containing asci and ascospores adapted as overwintering structure. Ascocarp is round to oval with irregularity arranged or scattered asci having dark brown to black colour and provided with appendages. Cleistothecium breaks open at maturity by wear and tear. e.g. Powdery mildew fungi of order Erysiphales.

4. Ascostroma

The asci formed directly in a locule or cavity within at stroma. The forms the wall of the ascocarp.

Basidiocarps

These are the fructification of sub-division, Basidiomycotina and consist of mushroom, bracket fungi, and puff balls. They are highly developed and have a compound structure, may be fleshy leathery woody waxy in nature and bear structures known as gills. The sexual spores known as basidiospores which are usually 4 in number. The basidia are intermingled with sterile structures called **paraphyses**.

1. Mushrooms

Mushrooms are the fleshy or leathery compound fruictification with variously coloured, commonly found on manure pits, dung heaps and on any rich organic matter. They are borne on stalk and provided with gills and pores to the underside which contains hymenial layer. The mushroom may be edible and non-edible or poisonous. e .g. *Agaricus* sp.

1. Puff balls

It is round or spherical basidiocarp , commonly found on dead organic matter. The basidiospores are produced in the hymenium which lines the inner surface. On maturity basidiospores are given off, in the form of puff or smoke.

2. Bracket Fungi

A compound fructification growing on dead tree trunks. These are woody and hard basidiocarp. They are typically bracket, hoof or saddle shaped and highly coloured. They are borne on short stalk. The hymenial layer is found on the honey comb fashioned pores in which basidia and basidiospores are observed.

Reproduction in Fungi

Reproduction

Reproduction is the formation of a progeny by either sexual or asexual means. Spore is an unit of reproductions.

Asexual Reproduction

This method of reproduction is characterized by production of identical individuals without the union of the sex organs.

Methods of Asexual Reproduction:

1. By fragmentation of soma or cell sap or hyphae
2. Budding
3. Binary fission
4. Production of spores

Sexual Reproduction

Sexual reproduction in fungi involves the union of two compatible nuclei.

Methods of Sexual Reproduction:

a. Planogamtic copulation
b. Gametangial contact
c. Gametangial copulation
d. Spermatization
e. Somatogamy
f. Heterokaryosis
g. Dikaryotization.

Asexual Reproduction of Fungi

1. By Fragmentation of Soma or Cell Sap or Hyphae

Fragmentation may also occur accidentally by the breaking off of parts of the mycelium through external forces. Such pieces of mycelium under favorable conditions can start a new individual. Laboratory propagation is frequently made from mycelial fragments.

2. By Arthrospores or oidia

The cells of the hyphae at the distal end round off and separate in basipetal succession. On germination , the arthrospores give rise to new fungus colonies.

3. By Chlamydospores

If the cells become enveloped in a thick wall before they separate from each other or from other hyphal cells adjoining the, they are called **chlamydospores**.

4. Budding

Budding is the asexual production of a small outgrowth from a parent cell. The bud increases in size while still attached to the parent cell. It eventually breaks off and forms a new individual . Sometimes chains of buds form a short mycelium. E.g. Rust and Smut fungi yeast fungi.

5. Binary Fission

Fission can occur through the simple splitting of a cell into two daughter cells by constriction. This is found among the bacteria generally, but some fungal yeasts may do this also.

6. Production of Spores

Spore produced may be conidia or sporangiospores basipetal oldest at the top and youngest at the bottom. Acropetal oldest at the bottom and youngest at the top.

Sexual Reproduction in Fungi

Sexual reproduction in fungi involves the union of two compatible nuclei. i.e. haploid.

Sexual Reproduction

The process of sexual reproduction consists of three distinct phases.

1. Plasmogamy

It is union of two protoplasts brings the nuclei close together within the same cell.

2. Karyogamy

Actual fusion of two haploid nuclei brought together as a result of plasmogamy , Karyogamy immediately follows plasmogamy.

3. Meiosis

The nuclear fusion is followed by meiosis. Meiosis reduces the number of chromosomes to haploid.

The sex organs in fungi are called as gametanigia, Gametangia from differentiated sex cells gametes or may contain one or more gamete nuclei.

Methods of Sexual Reproduction

a. **Planogametic copulation (Gametogamy):** This involves the fusion of two naked gametes one or both of which are motile. Motile gametes are called **planogametes.** Depending on the size and motility of the fusing gametes, there are three types

   Isogamy : Union of gametes that are similar in shape and size. e.g. *Synchytricum, Olpidium.*

   Anisogamy : Union of gametes that are morphologically similar but differ in size. e.g. Genus- Allomyces.

   Heterogamy: Union between a motile male gamete with a non motile female gamete is known as Heteroplanogametic copulation.

b. **Gametangial Contact:** In this method, two gametangia of opposite sex come in contact, and one or more gamete nuclei migrate from the male to the female. In no case do the gametangia actually fuse or in any way lose their identity during the sexual act. The male nuclei, in some species, enter the female gametangium through a pore developed by the dissolution of the gametangial walls at the point of contact; in other species, an especially developed fertilization tube serves as a passage for the male nuclei . After the passage of the nuclei has been accomplished the oogonium continues its development in various ways, and the antheridium eventually disintegrates. The zygote formed is called **Oospore**. e.g. Oomycetes , Ascomycetes.

c. **Gametangial Copulation:** Entire protoplast is transferred into the female gametangia a involes the fusion of two protoplast in a common cell. Sex gametes are indistinguishable or morphological identical. Copualtion occurs either by complete fusion of two protoplast. It is common in class Trichomycetes and zygomycetes.

d. **Spermatization:** It involves the formation of small spores or seed like structures or spematia. E.g. Spermatiospores. Spermatia acts as male gamete which is uninucleate or spore like and carried out by wind, insects to the retentive hypha (Female gametangium). A pore developed at the plant of contact and the contents of the spermatia passes into receptive hypha which serves as a female organ. e.g. Pycniospores and Receptive hypha in rusts.

e. **Somatogamy:** No gametes are involved. Vegetative hypha itself acts as a male and female gamete and bring about sexual reproduction. e. g. Smut Fungi.

f. **Dikaryotization:** Degenerate type of sexuality. It is accomplished through migration of nuclei from one cell to another cell of vegetative hypha, often through mechanism of clamps. The two nuclei remain in pair and divide as such and only fuse prior to the formation of spores. No special sex cells are produced. Clamp connections are formed during nuclear division. E.g. Class- Basidiomycetes.

g. **Heterokaryosis:** The phenomenon of the existence of genetically different kinds of nuclei in the same individual is called heteokaryosis (Gr. *heteros*=other + *karyon*=nut,nucleous), and the individuals that exhibit it are heterokaryotic. Heterkaryons may originate in a fungus thallus in four ways:

- By the introduction of genetically different nuclei into a homokaryon, a somatic cell in which all nuclei are similar.
- By the germination of a heterokaryotic spore, which will give rise to heterokaryotic soma.
- By mutation in a multinucleate, homokaryotic structure and the subsequent survival, multiplication, and spread of mutant nuclei among the wild type nuclei, and
- By fusion of some nuclei in a haploid homokaryon, and the subsequent survival, multiplication, and spread of the diploid nuclei among the haploid.

Special type of Sexual reproduction

Parasexuality: Some fungi do not go through a true sexual cycle as described. They may derive the benefits of sexual recombination through a process known as parasexuality.In this process, plasmogamy, karyogamy and haploidization take place, but not a specified points in the thallus or the life cycle. The parasxual cycle involves the following steps:

1. Formation of heterokaryotic mycelium
2. Nuclear fusion and multiplication of the diploid nuclei

3. Mitotic crossing over during the divison of the diploid cells.
4. Sorting out of the diploid strains.
5. Haplodization.

Taxonomy and Nomenclature Classification of Fungi

Taxonomy

Taxonomy is the science that deals with the identification nomenclature and classification of organisms.

Nomenclature

It is the system of assigning names to the taxonomic groups or organism according to international rules.

Systematics

It is scientific study of organisms with the ultimate object of characterizing and arranging them in an orderly manner.

Binomial System of Nomenclature

By Binomial system of nomenclature was developed by Carlous Von Linnaeus which is now universally used. As per the binomial system the name of organism is composed of two words.. The first word designates the genus and the genus name is always capitalized. The second word designates the species and its name is not capitalized. Binomials when written are underlined and when printed italicized. E.g. *Erwinia coli*, in which Erwinia is the genus and coli is the species.

Rules of Nomenclature

Following rules should be observed while righting of binomial.

1. The name of the genus should always be capitalized.
2. Species name should not be capitalized.
3. Binomial when written should always be underlined separately; when printed italicized.
4. The name or abbreviated name of the scientist describing the species for first time should be written after binomial. E. g. Pseudomonas syringae Val Hall.
5. If the name is revised, the name of the original describer should be written in bracket followed by the name of the revising scientist. E.g. *Xanthomonas compestris pv oryzae Dye.*
6. To avoid confusion the same binomial should not be used to name two different species.

7. The year in which organism was described should be written after the name of the author or scientist.

Sequence of Taxonomic Categories in Fungi

A sequence of taxonomic categories employed in the classification of microorganism is given below:

Taxa	Standard endings	Description
Super kingdom	Eukaryonta	------
Kingdom	Now Fungi	A group of similar divisions
Sub-kingdom	Mycota	----
Division	mycota (suffix)	A group of similar classes
Sub-division	mycotina (suffix)	----
Class	mycetes(suffix)	A group of similar orders
Sub-class	mycetidae (suffix)	-----
Order	ales (suffix)	A group of similar families
Family	aceae	A group or collection of similar genera
Genus	---	A group or collection of similar or closely related species.
Species	---	Collection of strains having similar Characteristics
Strain	----	It is population of organism that descends from a single organism or pure culture isolate.

Whittaker (1969) provided five kingdom system viz., Monera, Protista, Plantae, Animalia and Fungi, and thus Fungi is separated from Protista on the basis of nutrition pattern.

B. Natural and Artificial Classification

Natural classification: A natural classification attempts to place organisms in an orderly arrangement on the basis of overall resemblances, preferably on genetic basis. This classification reflect degrees of evolutionary relationships and therefore, may be phylogenetic.

Artificial classification: Classification based on one or few convenient characters to serve special purposes, e g. ease of identification, is called artificial classification.

C. Various classifications of Fungi

Classification of fungi was given by various authors viz. Gwynne-Vaughan and Barnes (1927), Martin (1931, 1941), E.A. Bessey (1950). C.J. Alexopoulos (1962) etc. The classification forwarded by Ainsworth (1966 and 1972) is most widely accepted that has been given below:

Kingdom : Protista (Fungi)

Sub-Kingdom : MYCOTA

1. Division : MYXOMYCOTA (Plasmodium or pseudoplasmodium are present)

Sub-division : Myxomycotina

Class : Acrasiomycetes
Class : Hydromyxomycetes
Class : Myxomycetes
Class : Plasmodiophoromycetes

2. Division: EUMYCOTA (Absence of Plasmodium or Pseudoplasmodium)

1. Sub-div : Mastigomycotina

Class : Chytridiomycetes
Class : Hyphochytridiomycetes
Class : Oomycetes

2. Sub-div : Zygomycotina

Class : Zygomycetes
Class : Trichomycetes

3. Sub-div : Ascomycotina

Class : Hemiascomycetes
Class : Plectomycetes
Class : Pyrenomycetes
Class : Discomycetes
Class : Laboulbaniomycetes
Class : Loculoasomycetes

4. Sub-div : Basidiomycotina

Class : Teliomycetes
Class : Hymenomycetes
Class : Gasteromycetes

5 Sub-div : Deuteromycotina

Class : Blastomycetes
Class : Hyphomycetes
Class : Coelomycetes

Subdivision: Mastigomycotina

General characters

- The Mastigomycotina includes all eumycota fungi which produce flagellated cells during their life cycle.

- Majority of them are with filamentous hyaline coenocytic mycelium.
- Cell wall contains cellulose.
- They show centric nuclear divison.
- The mode of nutrition is typically absorptive, because a majority of mastigomycotina contains some or other type of haustoria.
- They produce asexual spores called zoospores.
- Oospore is the sexual spores.
- Members of the class oomycetes are mostly aquatic but some are facultative or obligate parasites of vascular plants.

Classification

The Mastigomycotina consists of four classes

- Chytridiomycetes (with posteriorly uniflagellate zoospores)
- Hypochytridiomycetes (with anteriorly uniflagellate zoospores)
- Plasmodiophoromycetes (with anteriorly biflagellate zoospores)
- Oomycetes (biflagellate zoospores)

Class: Chytridiomycetes

- Characterized by the single posterior whiplash flagellum of their zoospores. It is divided into three orders

Order: Chytridiales

- True mycelium absent.
- Rhizomycelium present in some species.
- Fungi belonging to this order are only plant pathogenic.

Family: Olpidiaceae

Genus: *Olpidium*

Order: Blastocladiales

- True mycelium present.
- Sexual reproduction by planogametic copulation.
- Thick walled resting spore invariably formed.

Order: Monoblepharidales

- True mycelium present.
- Sexual reproduction by copulation between motile male and non motile female gamete contained in an oogonium (heterogametic copulation).
- No resistant sporangia.

Class: Plasmodiophoromycetes

Order: Plasmodiophoromycetales

Family: Plasmodiophoraceae

- All are obligate parasites of higher plants, algae and fungi.
- It form a wall less, naked **plasmodium** as the somatic phase.
- Plasmodium is a multinucleate mass of protoplasm, which can move in amoeboid fashion.
- It forms zoospores which bear two unequal flagella of whiplash type at their anterior end.

Genus: *Plasmodiophora*

Example: Club root disease of cabbage-*Plasmodiophora brassicae*

Class: Oomycetes

- The cell wall is made of cellulose.
- Zoospores biflagellate (posterior flagellum whiplash-type; anterior tinsel-type).
- In sexual reproduction the union of antheridia and oogonia produces oospores.

Order: Peronosporales

- Hyphae are well developed and aseptate.
- Cell wall is composed of glucan-cellulose complex and hydroxyproline.
- Parasites produce haustoria, which may be knob-like, elongated or branched and are found within the host cells.
- Asexual reproduction is by well-defined sporangia.
- Sexual reproduction is by means of well differentiated sex organs, antheridia (male) and oogonia (female).
- Oospores germinate directly or by producing a sporangium.

Family: Pythiaceae

- Sporangiophores similar to the vegetative hyphae or if different then of indeterminate growth.

Genus: *Pythium* and P*hytophthora*

The Difference between *Pythium* and *Phytophthora are given below*

S. No.	***Pythium***	***Phytophthora***
1	Hyphal wall contains greater amount of protein	Hyphal wall contains little amount of protein
2	Haustoria are absent	Haustoria are always present
3	Sporangiophores are indistinguishable from the somatic hyphae of the mycelium	Sporangia developed on specialized aerial hyphae, called sporangiophores.
4	Sporangia are either terminal or intercalary	Sporangia are always terminal
5	Zoospores are not differentiated inside the sporangium; undifferentiated sporangial contents are extruded into a vesicle in which the zoospores are differentiated	Zoospores are fully differentiated within the sporangium itself: vesicle is formed only rarely.
6	Appresoria are not formed	Appresoria may be formed
7	Sporangia are hyphal, spherical and rarely ovoid.	Sporangia are limoniform, obpyriform or ovoid

Important plant diseases caused by *Pythium* and *Phytophthora* spp. are

Fungus	**Disease**
Pythium	
Pythium debaryanum	Damping of tobacco and chillies
Pythium aphanidermatum	Soft rot of papaya, Damping off of potato
Pythium graminicolum	Rhizome and soft rot of turmeric
Pythium myriotylum	Foot rot of ginger
Phytophthora	
Phytophthora infestans	Late blight of potato
Phytophthora colocasiae	Colocasia blight
Phytophthora parasitica var. sesami	Leaf blight of Sesamum
Phytophthora palmivora	Bud rot of coconut palm and toddy palm

Family:Albuginaceae

- Sporangiophores strikingly different from vegetative hyphae, slender or thick, variously club-shaped, arranged in a layer, and bear sporangia in chain at the tip.
- These are obligate parasites.

Genus: *Albugo.*

Important plant diseases caused by *Albugo* spp. are

Fungus	**Disease**
Albugo candida	White blister on members of Cruciferae
Albugo bliti	White blister on members of Amaranthaceae
Albugo tragapogonis	White blister on members of Compositae
Albugo occidentalis	Infects Spinach

Family: Peronosporaceae

- Sporangiophores strikingly different from vegetative hyphae, Sporangia, singly or in clusters borne at the tip of characteristically branched sporangiophores of determinate growth.
- These are obligate parasites.

Classification of Peronosporaceae

Sclerospora	Pernospora	Plasmopara	Pseudoperonospora	Bremia
Sporangiophore is a long stout hypha, with many upright branches near the end, beraing sporangia at its tips	Sporangiophores are dichitomoulsy branched atacute angles and sporangia are borne on pointed tips.	Sporangiophoresare chotomously branched and sporangia are formed on short sterigmata and irregularly spaced.	Sporangiophores are dichotomously branched and sporangia germinate by means of zoospores.	Sporangiophores are dichotomously branched and tips of branches intocup shapedapophyses wih for sterigamata each bearing sporangia.
E.g. Downey mildew of bajara.-*S. graminicola*	E.g. Downey mildew of onion-*P.destructor*	E.g. Downey mildew of grape-*P.viticola*	E.g. Downey mildew of cucurbits - *P.cubensis*	E.g. Downey mildew of Lettuce-*B.lactucae*.

Order: Saprolegniales

- Zoospores are formed in zoosporangia.
- Oogonia never have a periplasm.
- A peculiar character of this group is the production of two types of zoospores in succession. This is called dimorphism or less accurately diplanetism.
- The two types of zoospores are termed primary and secondary zoospores.

Family: Saproleginaceae

Genus: *Saprolegina* and *Achlya*

The differences between *Saprolegina* and *Achlya* are given below:

Characters	**Saprolegina**	**Achlya**
Dimorphism	Present	Absent
Sporangial proliferation	Present	Absent
Zoospore liberation	Slow	In one stroke, the zoospores encysted at the tip of the sporangia to form a hollow ball of encysted, primary zoospores

Characters	**Saprolegina**	**Achlya**
Dimorphism	Present	Absent
Sporangial proliferation	Present	Absent
Zoospore liberation	Slow	In one stroke, the zoospores encysted at the tip of the sporangia to form a hollow ball of encysted, primary zoospores

Subdivision -Zygomycotina

General characters

- The majority of the members are saprobic. A few zygomycetes are weak parasites, attacking plants and animals.
- Most zygomycetes produce a well developed and branched mycelium, consisting of coenocytic hyphae.
- Cell wall is mainly composed of chitin.
- Motile cells or zoospores are absent.
- Asexual reproduction takes place by non motile sporangiospores called aplanospores.
- Sexual reproduction takes place by gametangial fusion.
- Gametangial fusion results in the production of a thick walled resting spore, called zygospore.

Class-Zygomycetes

Hasseltine and Ellis (1973) and a majority of the other workers divide zygomycetes into three orders.

(i) **Mucorales** : Chiefly saprophytic; asexual reproduction by spores or occasionally by conidia.

(ii) **Entomophthorales**: Chiefly parasitic on insects, asexual reproduction by modified sporangia acting like conidia or by true conidia. Modified sporangia are discharged with force.

(iii) **Zoopagales**: Chiefly parasitic on insects, asexual reproduction by modified sporangia acting like conidia or by true conidia. Conidia passively discharged.

Only Mucorales are discussed here.

Order: Mucorales

Family: Mucoraceae

Genus: Mucor and Rhizopus

The major difference between Mucor and Rhizopus are given below

S. No.	*Rhizopus*	*Mucor*
1	Rhizoids or holdfasts are present	Absent or less specialized
2	Stolons are present	Stolons are absent
3	Food material is absorbed mainly by rhizoids	Food is mainly absorbed by the entire mycelia surface
4	Sporangiophores develop in well organized groups mainly against the rhizoidal hyphae	Sporangiophores arise singly, and not in groups
5	Spores remain adhered to columella and are not easily disseminated	Spores easily blown away by wind
6	Most common Indian species is *R. stolonifer* (Sweet potato rot)	Some common species are *M. indicus, M.hiemalis, M.mucedo*

Subdivision: Ascomycotina, General characters

- Ascomycotina includes only such fungi in which the zygospores are absent and the perfect state spores are the ascospores.
- The Ascomycetes and Basidiomycetes are sometimes combindly called 'higher fungi'.
- Cell wall is made up of chitin.
- Mycelium is well developed branched and septate.
- Asexual spores are non-motile conidia.
- Sexual spores are ascospores.

- Ascospores are usually 8 in an ascus.
- They are produced endogenously inside the ascus.
- The asci are usually grouped to form a definite type of multicellular fruiting body called ascocarp.
- The ascocarps are either cup or saucer shaped (apothecium), flask shaped (perithecium), or closed, spherical and indehiscent (cleistothecium).
- The characteristic ascospores are present in sac- like body, called ascus and therefore these fungi are also commonly called 'sac fungi'
- Yeast is single celled organism.

Key to the classes of Ascomycotina

- Ascocarps and ascogenous hyphae absent, thallus yeast-like -**Hemiascomycetes**
- Ascocarps and ascogenous hyphae present, thallus mycelial: asci bitunicate, ascocarp an ascostroma - **Loculoascomycetes**
- Asci typically unitunicate, if bitunicate, ascocarp as apothecium: ascocarp a cleistothecium, asci evanescent and scattered - **Plectomycetes**
- Asci regularly arranged as basal or peripheral layer in the ascocarp Insect parasites - **Laboulbeniomycetes**
- Ascocarp perithecium, Not insect parasites, - **Pyrenomycetes**
- Ascocarp apothecium – **Discomycetes**

Class: Hemiascomycetes

- Characterized by the lack of ascocarp.
- Vegetative phase comprising of unicellular thallus or poorly developed mycelium.

It is divided into three orders

- **Endomycetales***:* Asci developing parthenogenetically from a single cell or directly from a zygote formed by population of 2 cells.
- **Taphrinales:** Asci arise from binucleate ascogenous cells formed by breaking of cells from hyphae.
- **Protomycetales:** Asci developing in a compound spore sac (syn ascus), produced singly from thick walled chlamydospores.

Order: Endomycetales

Family : Saccharomycetaceae

Genus:*Sacchromyces, Schizosaccharomyces,*

Fungus	Disease
Saccharomycetes cerevisiae	Brewer's and Baker's yeast

Order: Taphrinales

Family: Taphrinaceae

Genus: *Taphrina*

Fungus	Disease
Taphrina deformans	Leaf curl or leaf blister of peach
Taphrina maculans	Leaf spot of turmeric and ginger

Order: Protomycetales

Family: Protomycetaceae

Genus: *Protomyces*

Fungus	**Disease**
Protomyces macrosporus	Stem gall of coriander

Class: Loculoascomycetes

It comprises the following 5 ordcrs

Myriangiales, Dothideales, Pleosporales (Pseudosphaeriales), Hemisphaeriales (Microthyriales) and Hysteriales

Order: Myriangiales
Family: Myriangiaceae
Genera: *Elsinoe, Myriangium*

Order: Dothideales
Family: Capnodiaceae
Genera: *Capnodium, Limacinia*
Family: Dothideaceae
Genera: *Mycosphaerella, Guignardia*

Order: Pleosporales

Family: Venturiaceae

Genera: *Venturia*

Fungus	Disease
Venturia inaequalis	Apple scab

Class: Pyrenomycetes

- Characterized by unitunicate asci which arranged in a definite hymenium, usually inside a perithecium.
- The perithecia may be globose or flask shaped. In exceptional cases (Erysiphales- powdery mildews), the ascocarp may be a cleistothecium.
- Fungi having cleistothecia with a hymenium belongs to Pyrenomycetes.

Order: Erysiphales

Family: Erysiphaceae

It has the following genera.

1. Ascocarps present

A. Mycelium superficial

1. Ascocarp containing one ascus only
   a. Perithecial appendages simple, myceloid -*Sphaerotheca*
   b. Perithecial appendages dichotomously branched -*Podosphaera*
2. Ascocarp containing many asci
   a. Perithecial appendages simples, myceloid -*Erysiphe*
   b. Perithecial appendages coiled at the top –*Uncinula*
   c. Perithecial appendages dichotomously branched -*Microsphaera*

B. Mycelium partially endophytic

1. Perithecial appendages simple, imperfect state -Oidiopsis, *Leveillula*
2. Perithecial appendages coiled at the tip, imperfect state -Oidiopsis, –*Pleochaeta*
3. Perithecial appendages with basal swellings, imperfect state –*Ovulariopsis*

II. Ascocarp absent

A. Mycelium superficial

1. Basal cell of the conidiophores swollen
2. Basal cell of the conidiophores not swollen

a. Conidia borne in chains –*Euoidium*
b. Conidia borne singly –*Pseudoidium*

B. Mycelium partly endophytic

1. Conidia ovoid, obclavate -*Oidiopsis*
2. Conidia pyriform -*Ovulariopsis*

Order: Clavicipitales

Family: *Clavicipitaceae*

Genus: Claviceps

Fungus	**Disease**
Claviceps microcephala (C. fusiformis)	Ergot of pearl millet
Claviceps oryzae	False smut of rice
Claviceps purpurea	Ergot of rye
Claviceps sorghi (Sphacelia sorghi)	Ergot of sorghum

Powdery Mildews

- The fungi produces closed ascocarp called cleistothecium.
- The genera are differentiated based on the number of asci in the cleistothecium and type of appendages on it.
- Obligate parasites of higher plants mostly dicotyledons.

They are classified as follows.

I. One ascus in a cleistothecium

i. Myceloid appendages - e.g., *Sphaerotheca*
ii. Dichotomously branched appendages - e.g., *Podosphaera*

II. Many asci in a cleistothecium

i. Myceloid appendages - e.g., *Erysiphe, Leveillula.*
ii. Appendage coiled at the tip (circinoid type) - e.g., *Uncinula.*
iii. Dichotomously branched appendages - e.g., *Microsphaera*
iv. Appendage with bulbous base and spear like tip - e.g., *Phyllactinia*

Fungus	Disease
Powdery mildew of grapes	*Uncinula necator*
Powdery mildew of rose	*Sphaerotheca pannosa*
Powdery mildew of wheat	*Erysiphe graminis*
Powdery mildew of shisham	*Phyllactinia corylea*
Powdery mildew of wheat	*Erysiphe polygoni*
Powdery mildew of apple	*Podosphaera leucotricha*

Order: Meliolales

Family: Meliolaceae

Genus: *Meliola*

Class- Plectomycetes

- The asci are produced at different levels (not in a definite hymenium) inside the ascocarp, which is mostly a cleistothecium.
- The asci are unitunicate and evanescent (i.e. dehisce at maturity so that the ascospores lie free inside the cleistothecium.

Order: Eurotiales

Family: Eurotiaceae

Genus: *Aspergillus* and *Penicillium*

The Difference between *Aspergillus* and *Penicillium are given below*

S. No	*Aspergillus*	*Penicillium*
1	The conidiophores are aseptate and unbranched	The conidiophores are septate and branched
2	A conidiophores develops from a specialized thick walled cell, called foot cell	Foot cells are absent. Conidiophore develops from any vegetative cell of the mycelium.
3	Each conidiophores enlarges into a swollen vesicle at its tip	Vesicle are not formed
4	Metulae are not present	Metulae are present
5	Mature conidia are yellow, green, brown or black in colour	Usually the mature conidia are green in colour

Class-Discomycetes

- These are the Ascomycetes with apothecium type of fruiting bodies, which are cup shaped, saucer shaped or disc shaped.
- The shape of the ascocarp provides them the common name 'Cup fungi'.

Discomycetes are classified into seven orders. Only Pezizales and Tuberales are discussed here.

Order: Pezizales

Family: Pezizaceae (uninucleate ascospores present)

Genus: *Peziza*

Order: Tuberales

Family: Tuberaceae

Genus: *Tuber*

Subdivision -Basidimycotina

General characters

- The members are terrestrial, and saprophytic or parasitic.
- The mycelium is well developed, branched and septate. The mycelium is of primary, secondary and tertiary type.
- Dolipore septum is present except rusts and smuts.
- Clamp connections present.
- Cell wall consists of chitin and glucans.
- Basidiomycetes reproduce asexually by conidia, arthrospores, oidia, fragmentation or budding.
- No specialized sex organs develop in basidiomycetes.
- Plasmogamy takes place by somatogamy or spermatization.
- Sexual spores are basidiospores.
- They are exogenously produced on basidium.
- Usually four basidiospores are develop on basidium.
- The basidiomycotina includes rusts, smuts, mushrooms, jelly fungi, puffballs, shelf fungi, toadstools, bird's nest fungi, bracket fungi and earth stars.

Key to the classes of Basidiomycotina

- Basidiocarp lacking and replaced by teliospores grouped in sori or scattered within the host tissues - **Teliomycetes**
- Basidiocarp usually well-developed, Basidia typically organized as a hymenium; Saprobes or rarely parasites
  - Hymenium present and exposed before the spores mature. Basidiospores are violently discharged-**Hymenomycetes**
  - Basidiocarp remains closed at least until the basidiospores have been released from the basidia. Basidiospores not released with force; Basidium not involved in the discharge of spores.-**Gasteromycetes**

Class: Teliomycetes

- This class includes rusts and smuts.
- The class is characterized by thick walled, dikaryotic resting spores commonly called as teliospores in rusts and chlamydospores in smuts, Karyogamy takes place in this part and therefore, is actually a probasidium.

- The resting spores on germination produce promycelium (metabasidium) into which diploid nucleus moves and after meiosis four haploid nuclei are produced.
- These nuclei later, result in the formation of haploid basidiospores.
- Mycelial hyphae septate and the septa are of simple type.
- Asexual reproduction is uncommon, through dikaryotic spoes of conidial nature produced in rusts. In smut fungi, haploid sporidia may bud off into daughter cells.
- Basidiocarps absent.

This class is divided into 2 orders:

1. Uredinales

2. Ustilaginales

Order Uredinales (The rust fungi)

- These are obligate parasites and cause great losses to many cultivated crops.
- The mycelium is septate without clamp connections.
- It grows intercellularly, frequently producing haustoria.
- The rusts in which life cycle is short and completed by only two types of spores (teleutospores and basidiospores) are called microcyclic rust.
- The rust which has all the five spore stages (teleutospore, basidiospore, spermatia, pycniospore, aeciospore and uredospore) in its life cycle called macrocyclic rust.
- A macrocyclic rust in which uredospores are not formed has been named as demicyclic rust.
- The rust fungi that complete their life cycle in one host are termed as autoecious and those requiring two hosts for the completion of their life cycle are called as heteroecious.
- The rust fungi produce upto five types of spores in their life cycle, as given below:

Stage 0: Spermagonia with spermatia and receptive hyphae .

Stage I : Aecia with aeciospores

Stage II: Uredia with uredospores

Stage III: Telia with teleutospores

Stage IV: Basidia with basidiospores

(a) Pycniospores Stage(0)

- These are the spores produced in a flask-shaped structure called as pycnium, containing a palisade of sporogenous cells which produce spores in nectar exuded from the ostiole.
- Periphyses and flexuous hyphae (receptive hyphae) are commonly present in pycnia.
- Pycnia are formed in the host after it is infected by the basidiospores.
- Pycniospores are single celled and behave as spermatia.

(b) Aeciospores Stage (I)

- These are single celled dikaryotic spores produced in chains in cup-like structures known as aecia.
- The spores are yellow to orange in colour with a hyaline characteristically verrucose wall.

(c) Uredospores Stage (II)

- These are single celled binucleate, pedicellate deciduous spores borne in naked or paraphysate sori breaking through the host epidermis, commonly called as uredia or uredinia.
- Uredospores are brown, echinulate having almost conspicuous germ pores.
- They behave as conidia and repeat several cycles in a season and are also called as summer spores.

(d) Teliospores Stage (III)

- These are binucleate, pedicellate or sessile, erumpent or embedded in host tissue.
- They may be single celled, bicelled or more than 2-celled, with dark brown walls, having one or more germ pores.
- They produce basidium and basidiospores upon germination.

(e) Basidiospores Stage (IV)

- They are haploid, unicellular spores borne on sterigma.
- These arise from cylindrical to club-shaped 2 to 4 celled basidia.
- Depending on the reproductive stages present in the life cycle of rusts, rusts can be termed as 'macrocyclic'(all 5 stages present), 'demicyclic' (uredial stage absent) or 'microcyclic' (teliospore only as the binucleate spore).

- Rusts are either homothallic or heterothallic.
- In the former case pycnia, are not necessary and frequently absent.
- Dikaryotic phase starts from two cell nuclei at some point in the life cycle.
- In the case of heterothallic macrocyclic rusts, basidium bears four basidiospores; two of +type or two of -type.
- These basidiospores produce pycnia of + or-type respectively.
- The pycniospores behave as spermatia and fuse with the receptive hyphae of the opposite sex.
- The dikaryotic phase thus resulted, leads to the development of aecia.

Classification

There are four families in Uredinales

A. Teliospores pedicellate, germinating to form a promycelium, which become septate; spores uni -or multicellular, free - **Pucciniaceae**

B. Teliospores sessile

1. Teliospores in single, sessile, germinating to produce a septate promycelium; - **Melampsoraceae**
2. Teliospores in waxy crusts of one or two layers, becoming septate during germination without forming an external promycelium - **Coleosporiaceae**
3. Teliospores in chains - **Cronartianceae**

Family: Pucciniaceae

- The teliospores are pedicellate (Stalked).
- Teliospores are never present in the form of layers of crusts. They may be simple or compound .
- The uredinia may or may not have paraphyses.
- The aecia may be cup-like or naked.
- The peridium may be curved back.
- Spermagonia may be subcuticular and flattened or subepidermal and spherical with an ostiole.
- Both heteroecious and autoecious species are present.
- Other genera in Pucciniaceae are *Gymnosporangium, Phragmidium, Hemileia* and *Ravenelia.*

Classification

Important genera in Pucciniaceae are

1. Teliospores walls colourless; uredospores reniform, basidia slender, symmetrical ***-Hemileia***
2. Teliospore walls coloured, thickened, ornamented or with visible pores. Telia subepidermal, each pedicel bearing single teliospore. Pycnia subepidermal, globose; teliospore wall thicker above than sides or coloured or smooth ***-Uromyces***
3. Telia gelatinous, telial pedicel aseptate; teliospore cells arranged serially, with pedicel attached to the lower one only. On Cupressaceae - ***Gymnosporangium***
4. Teliospores not in fascicles. Pycnia globose, subepidermal; teliospores truly pedicellate, sometimes >2 celled - ***Puccinia***
5. Teliospore cells arranged as in phragmospores; teliospore wall coloured with 2 or more germ pores in each cell; pedicel usually long, teliospore without conspicuous outer hygroscopic layer - ***Phragmidium***
6. Teliospore cells arranged in a radially discoid head; teliospore pedicels several per head, fused together, telial head with hygroscopic cysts – ***Ravenelia***

Genus 1: *Puccinia*

- The genus Puccinia is an obligate parasite and is extremely host-specific.
- The teliospores are brown and are with mostly 2 cells.
- Telia are at first embedded in the host tissue but sooner or later the epidermis is ruptured and the spores become free. Spermagonia are subepidermal and spherical with ostiole.Aecia are cupulate with recurved peridium or maturity. Urediniospores (uredospores) are single and stalked, with long pedicel.
- They are often present in the same sori in which later the teliospores (teleutospores) are formed species are heteroecious.
- They mostly parasitize and cause rust diseases in Gramineae and Cyperaceae.
- Uredo- and teliospores are produced on wheat while spermatia and aeciospores are produced on barberry.
- The important plant pathogenic species are as follows:

Fungus	Disease
Puccinia recondita	Wheat brown or leaf rust
Puccinia graminis tritici	Wheat stem or black rust
Puccinia striiformis	Wheat yellow or stripe rust
Puccinia graminis hordei	Barley rust
Puccinia graminis avenae	Oat rust
Puccinia malvacearum	Holly hock rust
Puccinia arachidis	Groundnut rust
Puccinia asparagi	Asparagus rust
Puccinia helianthi	Sunflower rust
Puccinia hordei	Barley rust
Puccinia arachidis	Groundnut rust

Life cycle of *Puccinia*

There are three types of rusts based on the life cycle. They are

1. Macrocyclic rust
   a. Autoecious rust
   b. Heteroecions rust
2. Demicyclic rust
3. Microcyclic rust.

1. Macrocyclic rust: Five spore stages are produced in their life cycle.

a. Autoecious rust: Five spore stages are formed on a single host.

Examples:

- Linseed rust - *Melampsora lini*
- Sunflower rust - *Puccinia helianthi*
- Pea rust - *Uromyces fabae*
- Castor rust –*Melampsora ricini.*

b. Heteroecious rust: Two different hosts (*viz.*, primary host and alternate hosts) are required for completion of its life cycle.

- **Primary host** is the plant where the teliospores are produced.
- Alternate host is a plant which is required to complete life cycle without which the pathogen cannot survive.
- Uredia and uredospores and telia and teliospores are formed on the primary host.
- Pycnia and pycniospores and aecia and aeciospores are formed on the alternate hosts.
- Example: Wheat stem rust – *Puccinia graminis* var. *tritici.* For this rust wheat is the primary host and the barberry is the alternate host.

2. Demicyclic rust: Uredial stage absent and spermagonia may be present or absent.

Example- Cedar apple rust - *Gymnosporangium juniperi-virginianae*

3. Microcyclic rust: Teliospore is the only binucleate spore produced in this rust.

Example: Holly-cock *rust-Puccinia malvacearum.*

Genus: Uromyces

- It is characterized by the stalked, one celled teliospores on a simple pedicel with a papillum.
- Uredial, aecial and spermagonial characters are similar to *Puccinia.*
- The species may be heteroecious or autoecious.
- The important species causing pant diseases are given below.

Fungus	**Disease**
Uromyces ciceris-arietini	Gram rust
Uromyces *dianthi*	Carnation rust
Uromyces *fabae*	Vicia rust, lentil rust
Uromyces pisi	Pea rust

Family: Melampsoraceae

Genus: *Melampsora*

Fungus	Disease
Melampsora lini	Linseed rust
Melampsora ricini	Castor rust

Order: Ustilaginales

- The fungi included in this order are called smut fungi **.**
- Mycelium is intercellular and forms haustoria which draw nutrition from the host cells.
- Basidiospores are formed directly on a septate or non septate promycelium prodced by teliospores on germination.
- The teliospores are formed from all the cells of the secondary dikaryotic mycelium by developing a thick resistant wall.
- No sterigmata are formed. The sporidia develop directly on the promycelium.
- The basidiospores are discharge passively.
- Clamp connection and dolipore septum are generally absent.

- Barring one small family- Graphiolaceae, smuts donot form a basidiocarp

The differences between ustilaginalea and uredinales are given in the table below

Characters	Uredinales (rusts)	Ustilaginales (smuts)
Teliospores	Present, formed by terminal cells of secondary mycelium	Present,formed by intercalary as well as terminal cells of secondary mycelium
Basidiospores	Present in definite numbers, usually 4, borne on sterigmata; violently discharged	Not in definite numbers, Sterigmata absent; Basidiospores passively discharged,
Basidiocarp	Absent	Present in Graphiolaceae

There are two families in this order.

Family: Ustilaginaceae

- The family includes all the smut fungi in which the promycelium is transversely septate into several, usually four, cells with lateral and terminal sporidia, one or more from each cell. Sometimes there may be only one sporidium on the septate promycelium.
- Occasionally, the basidium (promycelium) develops directly into a mycelium without forming sporidia, as in *Ustilago nuda tritici,* or both conditions may be present (*Sphacelotheca sorghi*).
- Important genera are *Ustilago, Sphacelotheca*, *Tolyposporium* and *Melanopsichium*.

Ustilago

- Sori contain 1-celled teliospores, dusty at maturity and are covered by membrane of host origin.
- Germination is by means of septate promycelium, which may become infection hyphae or may produce sporidia laterally near the septa.
- The sporidia germinate easily in water by infection.
- The important species causing pant diseases are given below

Fungus	**Disease**
Ustilago nuda tritici	Loose smut of wheat
Ustilago zeae	Common smut of corn (syn. *U. maydis)*
Ustilago hordei	Covered smut of barley
Ustilago avenae	Loose smut of oats
Ustilago scitaminea	Whip smut of sugarcane

Family: Tilletiaceae

- The family includes only those smuts in which the promycelium is aseptate with terminal whorl of sporidia.
- The teliospores are single or combined into more or less permanent balls usually including sterile cells.
- Promycelium is simple, usually nonseptate up to the time of formation of sporidia.
- Sporidia are longer than in Ustilaginaceae, produced in clusters at the apex of the promycelium, fusing or not fusing in pairs, producing similar or dissimilar sporidia or germinating directly into infection threads.
- Important genera are *Tilletia, Neovossia, Urocystis, Entyloma* and *Turbicina*.

Class Hymenomycetes

- Well known mushrooms, jelly fungi, bracket fungi, toadstools, fairy clubs, tooth fungi, pore fungi, coral fungi and other similar forms are included under Hymenomycetes.
- This class is characterized by usually well-developed basidiocarp or fruiting bodies.
- The hymenium of the basidiocarps is fully exposed at maturity and consists of large number of basidia arranged in a palisade like manner.
- Basidiocarps are typically gymnocarpic (primordium and mature sporocarp have exposed hymenium) or semiangiocarpic (partially closed till spores are matured).
- Basidiospores are ejected forcibly i.e. these are ballistospores.

Classification

a. Basidia aseptate -Sub-class Holobasidiomycetidae.

b. Basidia septate -Sub-class Phragmobasidiomycetidae

Holobasidiomycetidae

- This class is characterized by an undivided, cylindrical to clavate basidium (i.e. holobasidum), which usually extends into four sterigmata each bearing a basidiospores.
- The basidia are produced in a well developed mycelium. Phragmobasidiomycetidae
- The metabasidium of these is completely or incompletely divided into 4 cells by transverse or longitudinal septa. The basidiocarp is usually gelatinous, waxy or dry.

- The probasidia may or may not be persistent.
- The basidiospores are often repetitive and sterigmata swollen.

Sub-class Holobasidiomycetidae

Order: Exobasidales

- The order is characterized by the 4-spored basidia, which form a layer (hymenium) on the leaf surface and lack the well-define basidiocarps.
- Consisting of the gall-forming plant parasites.

Family: Exobasidiaceae.

Genus; *Exobasidium*

Exobasidium vexans - blister blight of tea.

Order: Tulasnellales

Family: Ceratobasidiaceae

Genus: Ceratobasidium and Thanatephorus

Order: Aphyllophorales/ Polyporales

Family: Corticiaceae

Genera: *Chondrostereum, Peniophora, Athelia, Corticium*

Family: Ganodermataceae

Genus: *Ganoderma*

Order: Agaricales

- Commonly called 'gill fungi', which include mushrooms, (edible), toadstools (poisonous) and boletes.
- Mycelium of agaricales is typically basidiomycetous with primary, secondary and tertiary mycelia.
- The chracteristic macroscopic basidiocarp or fruit body is fleshy, generally having a stalk i.e. stipulate, and has a pileus bearing hymenium-covering lamellae on the underside.
- The young basidiocarp may be covered by a universal veil, which becomes broken down by the growth of the stipe and pileus but part may remain as volva at the base of the stipe and as fragments on the upper surface of the mature pileus.
- The developing hymenium may be covered by a partial veil, which later becomes a cortina or an annuals around the mature stipe.

- The hymenium may consist of cystidia of various kinds, setae, or hyphidia among the basidia the latter producing unicellular, hyaline or coloured ballistospores, typically in fours.
- Asexual reproduction is very rare. Only a few species show the production of thin walled oidia (*Coprinus lagopus*), chlamydospores (*Volvariella volvace(*a) or conidiophores as in members of Aphyllophorales.
- Sexual reproduction takes place by hyphal fusion and results in the formation of basidia and basidiospores, present together in the form of fruiting body , called basidiocarp.
- Except a few homothallic species, the majority of the members are heterothallic and show either unifactorial or bifactorial heterothallism.
- The order Agaricales contains 16 families (Smith, 1973). They are Boletaceae, Hygrophoraceae, Tricholomataceae, Entolomataceae, Amanitaceae, Pluteaceae, Lepiotaceae, Agaricaceae Bolbitiaceae, Strophariaceae, Coprinaceae, Cortinariaceae, Paxillaceae, Gomphidiaceae, Russulaceae and Cantharellaceae.

Family: Tricholomataceae

Genus: *Pleurotus,Armillariella, Marasmius*

***Pleurotus*:**

- This genus contains most valuable edible mushroom.
- Stripe is generally eccentric and pileus resupinate in some species. They have white or pigmented range fruiting bodies.
- They grow on wood, on dead or living hosts.

Pleurotus sajor -caju Oyster mushroom

Pleurotus ostreatus - Oyster mushroom.

Family : *Amanitaceae*

Genus: *Amanita,Limacella* and *Termitomyces*

Amanita

- The genus is characterized by free gills and the presence of the annulus and volva on the stripe.
- Remnant of the volva may persist as volva scales on the cap.
- More than 5 species are known to be mycorrhizal in habit.
- Some are more attractive and used in decoration. Some are poisonous and produce toxins called phallotoxin and amatoxins.

Amanita phalloides - Called 'Depth cap fungus'and it is poisonous.

Amanita virosa - called as 'Destroying angel'; or death angel and it is also poisonous.

Family: Pluteaceae

Genus: *Volvariella, Pluteus, Chamaeota.*

Volvariella

Volvariella volvacea and *Volvariella diplasia-* commonly called the straw, or paddy straw or Chinese mushrooms. are edible.

Family: Agaricaceae

Genus: *Agaricus, Cystoagaricus* and *Melanophyllium*

Agaricus

- The characteristic features of the genus are the presence of deep purplish brown free gills, and an annulus but no volva, and stalk that readily separates from the pileus.
- They are commonly found growing on ground in pastures.
- These mushrooms are edible for their delicacy.

A. campestris - White button mushroom; edible.

A. bisporus - edible and cultivated mushroom.

Edible mushrooms

- Mushroom is a fleshy to tough, edible umberella like basidiocarp (sporophores) of certain basidiomycetes fungi.
- The mushroom consists of stipe, a membranous annular ring called annulus, cap or pileus arid gills or lamellae.
- Each gill on cross section shows closely packed elongated fungal cells called trauma.
- A subhymenium with spherical cells is formed on both sides of the trauma.
- A fertile layer with palisade like cells called hymenium is found over the sub-hymenial layer
- It consists of club shaped basidia, sterigmata bearing single-celled basidiospores.
- In the hymenial layer stout sterile structure called cystidia are also found.
- The eating of mushrooms is called mycophagy

Morphology of Mushroom

- *Agaricus campestris* is a field mushroom growing on all organic matter in the fields.
- The mycelium is highly organized and the hyphae are often found to form rhizomorphs.
- Clamp connections are also formed by the hyphae and chlamydospores may be produced to resist the adverse conditions.
- The fruiting body or the basidiocarp commonly called as mushroom comes out of the soil and it consists of thick stalk called **stipe** on which an umbrella shaped **pileus**(cap) rest.
- The stipe is cylindrical in shape, fleshy and usually swollen at the base.
- Just above the middle the stipe has a membranous ring known as **annulus**.

The pileus on the under surface exhibits numerous structures radiating from the stipe. They are called **lamellae** or **gills**, which are slender, pink when young becoming brown later.

- The crosssection of a lamella or gills show the central loosely packed elongated fungal cells known as **trama**.
- On both sides of the trama are found **subhymenial** layers the cells of which will be spherical in shape. Over the sub-hymenial layer a layer of palisade-like cells known as **hymenial layer** is formed.
- The hymenial layer consist of club shaped **basidia** which have two to four minute **sterigmata** at their tip.
- The sterigmata bear the haploid single celled, ink basidiospores. In the hymenial layer there are some stout sterile structures known as **cystidia** (sing. cystidium).
- The **basidiospores** are released forcibly and fall near the base of the stipe and form a pink mass.

Agaricus

- *Agaricus* spp. are called button mushroom or **white button mushroom**.
- It has stout, cylindrical, fleshy umberella-like pileus and possess annulus.
- Good crop of mushroom comes at low temperature of 15 to 25° C.
- Well decomposed wheat / paddy straw compost incorporated with nutrients is used as substrate.
- The substrate mixture is filled in trays.

- The compost is now mixed with mycelial pieces(of the sixe of groundnuts) obtained from pure cultures of the fungus. This is called 'spawning. 'Hyphae permeate the compost.
- After 2-3 weeks the compost beds are covered with a thin layer, (2.5-3cm) of soil or peat-vermiculite mixture. This is called "casing".
- Without casing the fruiting bodies are not formed.
- The stimulating factor provided by the casing is not known.
- After amonth, fruiting bodies start making appearance.
- Higher temperature of the bed(15-21^{0}C) favour mycelia growth while a lower temperature (13-15^{0}C) favours fruiting body formation. So the temperature is kept below 15^{0}C after the initiation of fruiting.
- 300-350 kg of mushroom can be harvested from one ton of compost in a period of 85-100 days,
- It has two important commercia1 cultivated species

Agaricus bisporus -Temperate mushroom or white button mushroom,

Agaricus bitorquis- Hot weather mushrooms,

Pleurotus

- *Pleurotus* spp. are called oyster mushroom as it resembles shell of an oyster.
- The stipe is eccentric.
- It is called Dhingri in India.
- It is a tropical mushroom coming up well between 25-30°C.
- The colour may be white or grey or pink depending upon the species.
- It is grown on paddy straw (substrate) in polybags. In a period of 30-45 days, it yield 1.0 to 1.4 kg per kg of paddy straw.
- Commonly cultivated species in India are *Pleurotus sajor-caju, Pleurotus citrinopileatus, Pleurotus ostreatus, Pleurotus eryingii* etc.,

Subdivition: Deuteromycotina

General characters

- Deuteromycotina includes the fungi in which the 'perfect stage'(zygote, ascus, basidium) is either lacking or has not been discovered so far. Because of the apparent absence of any perfect stage or sexual phase, these fungi are commonly called 'imperfect fungi' or technically 'Fungi imperfecti'.

- The characteristic feature of Deuteromycotina is the absence of sexual reproduction. The members reproduce only be asexual methods, and that too also chiefly by conidia, which develop on conidiophores.
- The conidia are produced either directly on the conidiophores or in some special types of fruiting bodies such as synnemata, acervuli, sporodochia or pycnidia.
- Fungi possess branched, septate and multinucleate mycelium except the unicellular yeast like members of blastomycetes.
- Sexual reproduction is completely absent.
- Parasexuality is shown by some deuteromycotina. Under this phenomenon, the process of plasmogamy, karyogamy and haplodization take place, but not at specified time or specified points in the life cycle of the fungus.

Classification

The sub-divison Deuteromycotina is divided into following three classes:

1. **Blastomycetes:** True mycelium absent or not well-developed, soma is made up of yeast (budding) cells with or without pseudomycelium.
2. **Coelomycetes:** Mycelium well-developed, assimilative budding cells absent. Reproduction by conidia borne in pycnidia or acervuli.
3. **Hyphomycetes:** True mycelium is present; mycelium is either sterile forms o or bear spores on sporophores, which are never aggregated in pycnidia or acervuli.

Class: Hyphomycetes

- Majority of the members are either saprophytes or parasites.
- Mycelium well developed and septate.
- Majority of the genera reproduce by conidia (Moniliales), but some members reproduce only by fragmentation e.g. *Rhizoctonia* and *Sclerotium*.
- Neither pycnidia nor acervuli are produced by any member.

The class hyphomycetes is divided into following orders

Order

1. **Agonomycetales or Mycelial sterilia**: Conidia absent except for chlamydospores.
2. **Moniliales** : Conidia present, Conidiophores are not organized as synnemata or sporodochia- Conidiophores are organized as synnemata or sporodochia.
3. **Stilbellales:** Synnemata formed.
4. **Tuberculariales:** Sporodochia formed.

Order: Moniliales

- The conidiogenous cells are produced on the conidiophores, which may be either macronematous. i.e. which are morphologically very different from purely vegetative hyphae or micronematous. i.e morphologically similar to vegetative hyphae but are always mononematous i.e. they are sporodochia.
- The order is divided into four families, Moniliaceae, Dematiaceae and Stilbellaceae

Family 1: Moniliaceae

- The members of this form-family are characterized by the production of free conidiophores or conidiogenous cells from the somatic hyphae and all the structures i.e. hyphae.
- Conidiophores and conidia are hyaline or light coloured.

A key to important plant pathogenic genera is given here:

I. Conidia unicellular, globose to cylindrical, conidiophore distinct:

(a) Conidia almost similar to apical cells of conidiophores *Monilia*

(b) Conidia not as above; borne in chains; dry:

(i) Phialides in heads on simple conidiophores -*Aspergillus*

(ii) Phialides bush like; upright -*Penicillium*

(c) Conidia not borne in chains; conidiophores verticillate, phialospores in mucilaginous mass - *Verticillium*

(d) Conidiophore branching irregularly or dichotomously; conidia dry, borne on inflated apical cells -*Botrytis*

II. Conidia bicelled, ovoid to cylindrical:

(a) Conidiophores reduced to stromal cells - *Rhyncosporium*

(b) Conidiophoredistinct, rarely branched, in clusters; conidia cylindrical, in short chains - *Ramularia*

III. Conidia 3 or more celled

(a) Conidia usually of 2 types, multiseptate macroconidia sickle shaped; unicellular microconidia often present -*Fusarium*

(b) Conidiophores rarely branched, conidia simple, attenuated at the apex - *Cercosporella*

(c) Conidiophores usually simple; conidia on denticles –*Pyricularia Aspergillus* and *Penicillium.*

Family 2: Dematiaceae

- This family is characterized by the production of dark-conidia and/or conidiophores.
- Conidiophores are simple and not produced in any type of fruiting body.

Genera: *Alternaria ,Bipolaris, Cladosporium, Cercospora, Curvularia, Drechslera, Helminthosporium* and *Pyricularia.*

Alternaria

- It is a polyphagous fungus.
- Conidiophores are dark, septate, sometimes inconspicuous, simple or branched, bearing conidia at the apex.
- Conidia (Porospores) solitary or more often produced in acropetal succession to form simple or branched chains, muriform or dictyospore (transverse as well as longitudinal conidia, darkly pigmented, ovate to obclavate, tapering abruptly or gradually towards the apex, smooth or roughened.
- The perfect stage of *Alternaria* belongs to *Pleospora infectoria*

Important plant diseases caused by *Alternaria* spp. are

Fungus	Disease
Alternaria alternata	Black point disease of wheat
Alternaria brassicola	Leaf and pod spot of crucifers
Alternaria solani	Early blight of potato and leaf spot of tomato, chillies and tobacco
Alternaria porri	Purple blotch of onion
Alternaria brassicae	Leaf spot of crucifers
Alternaria triticina	Leaf blight of wheat

Cercospora

- *Cercospora* is characterized by long, hyaline or pigmented conidia borne in acropetal succession from a usually simple, sympodially extending, pigmented conidiophores which are frequently aggregated in fascicles .

- The conidia are long slender, narrow, tapering and contain many transverse septa.

Important plant diseases caused by *Cercospora* spp. are

Fungus	Disease
Cercospora arachidicola	Early leaf spot of groundnut
Cercospora personata	Late leaf spot of groundnut
Cercospora coffeicola	Leaf spot of coffee and spinach
Cercospora nicotianae	Frog -eye spot of tobacco
Cercospora kikuchii	Purple stain of soybean
Cercospora musae	Sigatoka disease of banana

Helminthosporium

- Mycelium immersed stromata usually present.
- Conidiophores often in fascicles, erect, brown to dark brown.
- Conidia develop laterally, often in verticils, through pores beneath the septa of the conidiophore while the tip of the conidiophores continues to grow but growth cases with the formation of terminal conidia.
- Conidia sub-hyaline to brown, usually obclavate, pseudoseptate and frequently with a dark brown to black protruding scar at the base.
- Colonies effuse, dark and hairy.
- *Helminthosporium* imperfect state is produced in *Pseudocochliobolus* belonging to the dothideales.

List of *Helminthosporium* transferred to *Drechslera*

***Helminthosporium* sp.**	***Drechslera* sp.**	**Ascigerous state**
Helminthosporium oryzae (Brown leaf spot of rice)	*Drechslera oryzae*	*Cochliobolus miyabeanus*
Helminthosporium maydis (Leaf blight of corn)	*Drechslera maydis*	*Cochliobolus heterosporus*
Helminthosporium gramineum (Leaf stripe of Barely)	*Drechslera graminea*	*Pyrenophora graminea*
Helminthosporium sativum (Leaf blight of wheat)	*Bipolaris sativum*	*Cochliobolus sativum*

Drechslera

- Drechslera is characterized by the sympodially extending conidiophore, which produces an acropetal succession of multiseptate porospores, which are cylindric in shape and germinate from any or all cells.

- Conidiophores are indeterminate, extending by sympodial growth, brown and produce the conidia singly at the apices.
- Conidia are cylindrical, multiseptate and dark.
- *Cochliobolus, Pyrenophora, Pleospora* and *Trichometasphaeria* are imperfect states of *Drechslera.*

Bipolaris

- It is characterized by germination of conidia from the end cells only.
- Conidiophores brown, producing conidia through an apical pore and forming a new apex by growth of the sub-terminal region.
- Conidia fusoid, straight or curved, germinating by one germ tube from each end cell.
- The perfect state is *Cochliobolus*.

Pyricularia

- Conidiophores are more or less erect, simple or rarely branched, septate, hyaline to lightly pigmented.
- Conidia borne singly and terminally at the apex of conidiophore with successive conidia being produced in acropetal succession.
- Conidia ellipsoid or more often pyriform, broader and truncated at the attachment point, tapering towards the distal end, mostly one septate or two septate, hyaline to lightly pigmented.

Important plant diseases caused by *Pyricularia* spp. are

Fungus	Disease
Pyricularia oryzae	Blast of rice
Pyricularia setare	Blast of fox-tail millet
Pyricularia grisea	Blast of ragi / Finger millet

Curvularia

- Conidiophores are erect, macronematous and mononematous.
- The conidia develop either spirally or in whorls on conidiophores.
- The conidia are usually curved.
- Usually the third cell from the base of the conidium is largest.

Example: *Curvularia cambopogonis*

Family 3: Stilbellaceae

- Conidia and conidiophores develop in synnemata.

Genus: *Graphium*

Order: Tuberculariales

- The characteristic features of this order is the production of sporodochia.

Family: Tuberculariaceae

Genera. *Fusarium*

- The macroconidia (phialospores) are produced on conidiophores, which may be solitary and simple or aggregated (sporodochi(a) and with complex branching and the ultimate branched terminating in sporogenous cells.
- Microconidia are non-septate or one-septate, ovoid to short cylindric, gathering in short chains or more commonly in spore balls.
- Thick walled chlamydospores are also produced either terminally or intercalarily on the somatic hyphae.
- The mycelium, microconidia, macroconidia and sporodochia are bright in colour.
- Perfect state of *Fusarium* is found in Ascomycetes in the family Hypocreaceae in which the genera, *Nectria, Calonectria, Gibberella* and *Micronectriella* are found.

Important plant diseases caused by *Fuarium* spp. are

Fungus	Disease
Fuarium moniliforme	Foot rot of rice
Fuarium oxysporum f.sp. *batatae*	Wilt of sweet potato
Fuarium oxysporum f.sp. *coriandri*	Wilt of coriander
Fuarium oxysporum f.sp. *cubense*	Panama disease of banana
Fuarium oxysporum f.sp. *glycines*	Wilt of soybean
Fuarium oxysporum f.sp. *lagenariae*	Wilt of bottlegourd
Fuarium oxysporum f.sp. *lathyri*	Wilt of *Lathyrus sativus*
Fuarium oxysporum f.sp. *lentis*	Wilt of lentil
Fuarium oxysporum f.sp. *lini*	Wilt of linseed
Fuarium oxysporum f.sp. *lycopersici*	Wilt of tomato
Fuarium oxysporum f. sp. *Melongenae*	Wilt of brinjal
Fuarium oxysporum f.sp. *pisi*	Wilt of pea
Fuarium oxysporum f. sp. *psidii*	Wilt of guava
Fuarium udum	Wilt of pigeonpea

Class: Coelomycetes

- The thallus is eucarpic, mycelia and septate.
- Conidia are produced either in acervuli or pycnidia.
- The conidia are unicellular, deciduous and hyaline or pigmented.
- Coelomycetes is divided into two orders, Melanconiales and Sphaeropsidales.
    1. Melanconiales: Conidia produced in acervuli
    2. Sphaeropsidales: Conidia produced in pycnidia

Order: Melanconiales

- The fructifications are acervuli. It contains a single family.

Family: Melanconiaceae

- Characterized by the production of acervuli.
- Conidia may be hyaline to cream, pink, orange or black.
- They cause plant disease known as anthracnose.
- The important genera are *Colletotrichum, Cylindrosporium, Melanconium, Pestalotia, Pestalotiopsis, Gloeosporium*

Colletotrichum

- Acervuli may be subcuticular, epidermal or subepidermal.
- Conidiophores are hyaline to brown, septate, smooth, branched at the base.
- Conidia are hyaline, unicellular, falcate or lunate (sickleshaped) or cylindrical.
- Perfect state of the fungus belongs to *Glomerella.*

Important plant diseases caused by *Colletotrichum* spp. are

Fungus	Disease
Colletotrichum capsici	Fruit rot and dieback of chillies, Anthracnose and boll rot of cotton.
Colletotrichum graminicola	Anthracnose of corn and sorghum
Colletotrichum circinans	Smudge of onion
Colletotrichum falcatum	Red rot of sugarcane
Colletotrichum gloeosporioides	Anthracnose of citrus and banana.
Colletotrichum lindemuthianum	Anthracnose of cowpea
Colletotrichum musae	Anthracnose of banana
Colletotrichum coffeanum	Anthracnose of coffee

Pestalotia

- The genus is characterized by the conidia which are fusiform, straight or slightly curved and five septate.
- There may be 3-9 apical, cellular, simple or dichotomously branched appendages and one basal endogenous cellular, simple or branched appendage.
- The conidiophores are long, branched and septate.
- The fructifications are dark brown.

Important plant diseases caused by *Pestalotia* spp. are

Fungus	Disease
Pestalotiopsis palmarum	Grey blight of coconut.
Pestalotia theae	Grey blight of tea and blight of mango, palms and cotton.
Pestalotia mangiferae	Grey blight of mango.

Order: Sphaeropsidales

- The conidia and conidiophores are produced in pycnidia.
- Mycelium may be immersed in the substrate or superficial.
- Conidia are solitary, sympodial catenate etc.
- Sphaeropsidales is divided into four families based on the colour, shape and texture of the pycnidia.
- They are Sphaeropsidaceae ,Nectrioidaceae, Leptostromataceae and Excipulaceae

Family : Sphaeropsidaceae

- This is a large family consisting of both saprobes and a stroma.
- The spores are hyaline spherical or oval and often exude from the ostiole in damp weather in a worm like mass or citrus.

Macrophomina

- Mycelium superficial or immersed, hyaline to brown, branched, septate.
- Pycnidia separate, globose, dark brown, immersed, with one cavity, thick walled.
- Ostiole central, circular, papillate.
- Conidiophores absent.
- Conidia (Pycnospores) hyaline, aseptate, obtuse at each end straight cylindrical to fusiform.

- Forming mainly sclerotia in cultures, which are black, smooth, hard, formed of dark-brown thickwalled cells.

Genus: *Macrophomina*

Important plant diseases caused by *Macrophomina* spp. are

Fungus	Disease
Macrophomina phaseolina (syn. Rhizoctonia bataticola)	Charcoal rot, Ashy stem blight, Dry root rot, Canker, Damping off and leaf lesions on hosts like soybean, groundnut, cotton,

Ascochyta

- Mycelium immersed, branched, septate, hyaline to pale brown.
- Pycnidia are amphigenous, separate, globose, brown, immersed, unilocular and thin-walled.
- Ostiole central, circular, slightly papillate.
- Conidiophores are absent.
- Conidia hyaline, thin-walled, cylindrical, ovoid, oblong to irregular, medianly one-septate, continuous or constricted at the septum.
- Conidia may be guttulate.

Important plant diseases caused by *Ascochyta* spp. are

Fungus	**Disease**
Ascochyta abelmoschi	Leaf, fruit and stem spot of lady's finger.
Ascochyta carica	Fruit rot of papaya
Ascochyta fabae	Leaf and pod spot of broad beans
Ascochyta phaseolorum	Leaf and pod spot of common bean and other legumes.
Ascochyta pisi	Leaf and pod spot of pea
Ascochyta rabiei	Blight of chickpea
Ascochyta sorghi	Leaf spot of sorghum

Septoria

- The pycnidia are immersed in the substratum and are either separate or aggregated .
- They are globose, ostiolate, thin walled and brown.
- Conidia are hyaline, smooth, filiform, continuous or constricted at septa.
- The perfect states in Ascomycotina genera are *Mycosphaerella* and *Leptosphaeria*.

Important plant diseases caused by *Ascochyta* spp. are

Fungus	**Disease**
Septoria apii	Celery leaf blight
Septoria bataticola	Leaf spot of sweet potato
Septoria glycinea	Brown spot of soybean
Septoria lycopersici	Leaf spot of tomato
Septoria nodorum	Speckled leaf blotch of wheat
Septoria tritici	Leaf spot of wheat

Family: Excipulaceae

Genera: *Excipula, Discula, Dinemosporium, Sporonema*

Order: Agonomycetales or Mycelia sterilia

Genus: *Rhizoctonia* and *Sclerotium.*

Rhizoctonia

- They are facultative necrotrophs i.e. they are capable of prolonged existence as saprophyte in the soil.
- They form sclerotia of irregular size and shape but of uniform texture brown or black, more or less loosely packed.
- The cells of the hyphae are barrel shaped, anastomosing frequently, branching more or less at right angles, and pale brown to brown in colour.
- Perfect states of *Rhizoctonia* are *Ceratobasidium* and *Thanatephorus* (of Basidiomycotin(a) and *Macrophomina* (Pycnidial state).

Important plant diseases caused by *Rhizoctonia* spp. are

Fungus	Disease
Rhizoctonia bataticola	Dry root rot of pulses, cotton etc. (Pycnidial state: *Macrophomina phaseolina)*
Rhizoctonia solani	Root rot of cotton. (Perfect state: *Thanatephorus cucumeris)*

Sclerotium

It is characterized by hard, brown to black, fairly large sclerotia. These are produced on sterile, cotton, white mycelium provided with clamp connections.

The perfect states of *Sclerotium* are *Pellicularia* (Hymenomycetes of Basidiomycotina) and (*Sclerotinia* of Ascomycotina)

Important plant diseases caused by *Sclerotium* spp. are

Fungus	Disease
Sclerotium cepivorum	White rot of onion
Sclerotium rolfsii	Root rot of soybean, black pepper groundnut, cotton, cabbage tomato etc
Sclerotium oryzae	Stem rot of rice

Teleomorphic stage of some Important Pathogens

S. No	Anamorphic stage	Teleomorphic stage
Cleistothecial ascomycetes		
1	*Penicillium*	*Talaromyces*
2	*Oidium*	*Erysiphe*
3	*Paecilomyces*	*Byssochlamys*
4	*Aspregillus*	*Eurotium*
	Perithecial ascomycetes	
5	*Colletotrichum*	*Glomerella*
6	*Fusarium*	*Gibberella*
7	*Trichoderma*	*Hypocrea*
8	*Verticillium*	*Hypocrea*
9	*Graphium*	*Ophiostoma*
10	*Chalara*	*Ceratocystis*
11	*Acremonium*	*Epichloe*
	Loculoascomycetes	
12	*Alternaria*	*Lewia*
13	*Cercospora*	*Mycosphaerella*
14	*Septoria*	*Mycosphaerella*
15	*Phyllosticta*	*Guignardia*
16	*Stemphylium*	*Pleospora*
17	*Bipolaris*	*Cochliobolus*
18	*Drechslera*	*Pyrenophora*
19	*Exserohilum*	*Setosphaera*
20	*Curvularia*	*Cochliobolus*
21	*Sphaeropsis*	*Physalospora*
		Apothecial ascomycetes
22	*Monilia*	*Monilinia*
23	*Botrytis*	*Botryotinia*
24	*Melanconium*	*Greeneria*
25	*Cylindrosporium*	*Myocspharella*
26	*Entomosporium*	*Diplocarpon*
		Basidiomycetes
27	*Rhizoctonia*	*Thanatephorus*
28	*Sclerotium*	*Aethalium*

Model Practice Questions

A. Objective Questions

a. Multiple Choice Questions

1. The mass of hyphae constitute the fungus thallus is
   (a) Mycelium (b) Stroma
   (c) Rhizomorph (d) Prosenchyma
2. The non-motile spores are known as
   (a) Zoospores (b) Aplanospores
   (c) Planospores (d) Oospores
3. Union of gametes of fungi that are similar in shape and size is called
   (a) Isogamy (b) Anisogamy
   (c) Heterogamy (d) None
4. The structure help in survival to fungi under adverse conditions is
   (a) Sclerotia (b) Chlamydospore
   (c) Oospore (d) All the these
5. The zoospore production is absent in
   (a) Albugo (b) Phytophthora
   (c) Pythium (d) Rhizopus
6. A pore like opening in perithecia and pycnia through which spores escape from fruiting body is
   (a) Ostiole (b) Haustorium
   (c) Hole (d) Paraphysis
7. Formation of coenocytic mycelium is the feature of
   (a) Oomycetes (b) Ascomycetes
   (c) Basidiomycetes (d) Zygomycetes
8. Zoospore having a single posterior whiplash flagellum is produced by
   (a) Oomycota (b) Chytridiomycota
   (c) Zygomycota (d) Ascomycota
9. Fungi forming vesicular- arbuscular mycorrhizae come under the order
   (a) Glomales (b) Mucorales
   (c) Hypocreals (d) Helotiales

10. Fungus forming vesicular- arbuscular mycorrhizae is

(a) Glomus (b) Acaulospora
(c) Gigaspora (d) All of the above

11. Gibberella spp. is a

(a) Cleistothecial ascomycetes (b) Perithecial ascomycetes
(c) Loculoascomycetes (d) Apothecial ascomycetes

12. Elongated non-septate mycelium, biflagellate zoospores and oospore production is the feature of

(a) Mycota (b) Myxomycetes
(c) Chytridiomycetes (d) Zygomycetes

13. The 'division' ends up with

(a) Mycot (b) Mycotina
(c) Mycetes (d) Mycetidae

14. Genera like-Ustilago, Urocystis, Nevossia and Tolyposporiusm come under the order

(a) Ustilaginales (b) Uredinales
(c) Exobasidiales (d) Agaricales

15. Vascular wilt causing pathogen is

(a) Fusarium and Verticillium (b) Erwinia and Ralstonia
(c) Pythium (d) All of the above

16. Conidia with cross walls on both axes is the identification character of

(a) Alternaria (b) Stemphylium
(c) Capnodium (d) All of the above

17.Closed ascocarp is

(a) Perithecium (b) Cleistothecium
(c) Apothecium (d) Ascostromata

18. The cell wall of oomycetes contain

(a) Chitin (b) Cellulose
(c) Chitosan (d) All of these

19. Spore bearing hypahe is

(a) Sporangiophore (b) Conidiophore
(c) Sterigmata (d) Conidiomata

20. The existence of a number of races or forms of one species of pathogen is
    (a) Physiological specialization (b) Ecological specialization
    (c) Biochemical specialization (d) Ontogenic specialization

21 The fungi which transmit plant viruses belong to class–
    (a) Basidiomycetes (b) Oomycetes
    (c) Zygomyctes (d) Plasmodiophoromycetes

22.'Buller's phenomenon" is associated with
    (a) Ascomycetes (b) Basidiomycetes
    (c) Deuteromycetes (d) Zygomycetes

23. Chocking of vascular bundles by fungal hyphae is observed in
    (a) Root rots (b) Wilts
    (c) Anthracnose (d) Downy mildew

24.An open, cuplike, or saucer-shaped sexual fungal fruiting body containing asci.
    (a) Apothecia (b) Perithecia
    (c) Cleistothecia (d) Pseudothecia

25 The fruiting body presents in Claviceps fungi
    (a) Apothecia (b) Perithecia
    (c) Cleistothecia (d) Pseudothecia

26.The Ascomycetes and Basidiomycetes are sometimes combindly called '
    (a) Higher fungi (b) Lower fungi
    (c) Medium fungi (d) All

27. The fruiting body presents in Erysiphe fungi
    (a) Apothecia (b) Perithecia
    (c) Cleistothecia (d) Pseudothecia

28. The fruiting body presents in *Peziza* fungi
    (a) Apothecia (b) Perithecia
    (c) Cleistothecia (d) Pseudothecia

29. The Basidiomycotina includes
    (a) Rust (b) Smut
    (c) Mushrooms (d) All

30. The pedicellate teliospore present in family
    (a) Pucciniaceae (b) Melampsoraceae
    (c) Coleosporiaceae (d) Cronartianceae

Sl. No	Answer	Sl. No	Answer
1	(a) Mycelium	16	(a) Alternaria
2	(b) Aplanospores	17	(b) Cleistothecium
3	(a) Isogamy	18	(b) Cellulose
4	(d) All the these	19	(a) Sporangiophore
5	(d) Rhizopus	20	(a) Physiological specialization
6	(a) Ostiole	21	(d) Plasmodiophoromycetes
7	(a) Oomycetes	22	(b) Basidiomycetes
8	(b) Chytridiomycota	23	(b) Wilts
9	(a) Glomales	24	(a) Apothecia
10	(d) All of the above	25	(b) Perithecia
11	(b) Perithecial ascomycetes	26	(a) Higher fungi
12	(a) Oomycetes	27	(c) Cleistothecia
13	(b) Mycota	28	(a) Apothecia
14	(a) Ustilaginales	29	(d) All
15	(a) Fusarium and Verticillium	30	(a) Pucciniaceae

b. True/False

1. Fungi are eukaryotic, spore bearing, achlorophyllus, heterotrophic, thallophytic plants.
2. Cell wall of fungus is well defined, typically made up of cellulose.
3. Appressoria are localized swellings of the tip of germ tube that develop in response to contact with the host.
4. The organized fungal tissues are called Plectenchyma.
5. Plasmogamy is union of two protoplasts brings the nuclei close together within the same cell.
6. Somatogamy found in smut fungi .
7. Binomial system of nomenclature was developed by Carlous Von Linnaeus.
8. The perfect state present in zygomycotina is Ascospore.
9. The class oomycetes has biflagellate zoospores.
10. The genus Albugo is an obligate parasites.
11. Saprolegina show a peculiar character of diplanetism.
12. The fruiting body ascocarps is cup or saucer shaped apothecium.
13. The class discomycetes possess apothecium type of ascocarp.
14. Perithecial appendages coiled at the top in the genus Uncinula.
15. The fructifications acervuli are found in Colletotrichum.

16. The conidia and conidiophores develop in synnemata in genus Graphium.
17. Deuteromycotina includes the fungi in which the 'perfect stage'is present.
18. The telemorphic stage of Colletotrichum is Glomerella.
19. The anamorphic stage of Lewia is Alternaria.
20. The telemorphic stage of Rhizoctonia is Thanetophorus

Question. No	Answer	Question No	Answer
1	True	11	True
2	False	12	True
3	True	13	True
4	False	14	True
5	False	15	True
6	True	16	True
7	True	17	False
8	False	18	True
9	True	19	Yrue
10	True	20	True

B.Descriptive Questions

a. Short Answers

1. Why the genus written with an initial capital letter and species with small letter.
2. Write the standard endings for various taxa of fungi, starting from phylum. Which taxa donot have standard endings?
3. Short notes
   a. Write names of five catastrophic diseases of plants.
   b. Name the kingdom of fungi.
4. Elaborate the similarities and differences between the various kingdoms of fungi.
5. Which is the authentic publication on taxonomy of fungi?
6. Why deutermycotina is called fungi imperfecti?
7. Write down the differences between rust and smut.
8. Classify order erysiphaes with suitable examples.

b. Long Answers

1. What is fungus? Write down their general characters and method of reproduction.
2. Discuss in details about sexual and asexual reproduction in fungi.
3. What is fungi? Write down the characters of fungi.
4. Write short notes on
   i. Parasexuality
   ii. Heterokaryosis
   iii. Dikaryotization
   iv. Fungal tissue.
5. Differentiate between
   (a) Haustoria and Appresoria
   (b) Homothallic fungi and Heterothallic fungi
   (c) Gametangial contact and Gametangial copulation
   (d) Cytokinesis and Karyokinesis
6. Differentiate between
   1. Sexual reproduction and Parasexual reproduction
   2. Isogamy and Anisogamy
   3. Spermatization and Somatogamy
   4. Rhizomorph and Sclerotium
7. Explain the major classifications of fungi and the characteristics of each group.
8. Describe the characteristics of the Ascomycota group and its significance in both ecology and human life.
9. Compare and contrast Zygomycota and Ascomycota, focusing on their structural and reproductive differences.
10. Discuss the importance of fungi in the nitrogen cycle and other ecological processes.
11. What is the role of Deuteromycota in the classification of fungi, and why is it considered an artificial group?

10

Bacteria Morphology, Reproduction Classification of Phytopathogenic Bacteria

Definition

Bacteria belong to proakaryota which encompasses organisms with a primitive type of nucleus lacking a clearly defined membrane .The bacteria are smaller than fungi and measure about 0.5 to 1.0 x 2.0 to 5.0μ.

Structure of bacteria

1. A bacterial cell consists of a cell wall and a compound membrane enclosing protoplasm.
2. The protoplasm contains the nucleus, vacuoles, mesosomes, lipids, polysaccharides, mitochondric granules, and spores.
3. Bacterial cells may have flagella, pili, fimbrae, and capsules on the outside.
4. The bacterial cell contains a characteristics cell wall. The cell wall of bacteria is composed of a peptidoglycan. It is composed of acetyle-glucosamine and cetyle-muramic acid .
5. The rigid peptidoglycan layer is located between the cytoplasmic membrane and an outer multiple tract layer.
6. The latter layer is composed of lipoprotein . It is common in gram negative bacteria.
7. Many bacteria possess other intracellular membrane systems such as mesosomes and chondrioids.
8. The mesosome structure is formed by an invagination of the cytoplasmic membrane.
9. Mesosomes serve for compartmentalization and integration of biochemical systems.

10. The cell material contained within the cytoplasmic membrane can bedivided into the cytoplasmic are rich in RNA , nuclear area rich in DNA and the fluid portion with dissolved nutrients.
11. Bacteria do not have characteristic nucleus. They contain bodies within the cytoplasm that are regarded as a nuclear structure and DNA is confined to this area.
12. Bacteria contain 3 to 70 ribosomes depending upon the bacteria. Ribosomes are the sites of protein synthesis.
13. Lipids are found in the cytoplasm of bacteria in the form of fat globules.
14. Glycogen accumulates in the cytoplasm at the ends of the cell in the form of granules.
15. Some of the bacteria possess flagella which are useful for motility of the bacteria.
16. The bacteria belonging to eubacteriales have peritrichous flagellus-flagella at all the sides.
17. Some bacteria transform themselves into small ovals or spheres which are highly resistant to adverse conditions. They are called as spores.
18. Bacterial spores have dipicolinic acid which is absent in vegetative cells. Dipicolinic acid is found only in bacterial spores.
19. Fibriae are hair like structures that are observed as surface appendages on some bacteria. Fimbriae are common in plant pathogenic bacteria.
20. Pili are also hair like structures found in some bacteria. They serve as adsorption organs for bacteriophages. Pili mediate conjugation of bacteria.
21. Most of the plant pathogenic bacteria are rod shaped except *Streptomyce*s which are mostly filmentous.
22. Majority of plant pathogenic bacteria are aerobic except; *Erwinia.*
23. Plant pathogenic bacteria required optimum growth temperature ranging between 27-30^{0}C.
24. Most of the plant pathogenic bacteria reproduce by asexual process known as binary fission or fission.
25. Most of the plan pathogenic bacteria are gram negative except *Streptomyces, Clavibactor, Curtobacterium, Nocardia* and *Rhodococcus* which are gram positive in Gram's reaction.
26. In *Streptomyces, Clavibacter* and *Bacillus* a part of cell membrane envaginates into the cytoplasm to form complex membrane infolding called as mesosomes.

27. .*Bacillus* and *Clostridium* species produce endosproes which are dormant structures.
28. Bacterial cell lacking cell wall is called protoplast.
29. The naked protoplast may synthesize a portion of cell wall material. Such a protoplast is called sphaeroplast.
30. L forms are non rigid bacterial forms. They are soft protoplasmic elements without defined morphology which can be propagated indefinitely on solid medium.
31. L-form of bacteria are usually produced under unfavourable conditions or in laboratory when penicillin or other substances that inhibit cell wall production are added to culture medium.
32. The L-form plant pathogenic bacteria reported are *Agrobacterium tumefaciens* and *Erwinia.*
33. Protoplast, sphaeroplasts and L-forms are all bacterial forms devoid of the rigid cell wall.
34. Plasmids are extra chromosomal DNA capable of autonomous replication. Some bacteria have plasmids in the cytoplasm. They are not capable of integrated with the chromosome.
35. Episomes are similar to plasmids. They are also autonomous and dispensable genetic elements. But unlike plasmids, episomes, can exist even integrated with the chromosome.
36. Generally the bacteria contains plasmids do not have episomes and vice versa.
37. Transposons are mobile DNA segments that can insert into afew or several sites in a genome .
38. Transponsons are even capable of moving between prokaryotes and eucaryotes.
39. Siderophores are produced by many bacateria extracellularly. They are low molecular weight iron (III) transport agents. The function of siderophores is to supply iron to the cell.The siderophore isolated from *Pseudomonas* sp. is called **pseudobactin.**
40. Bacteriosins are non replicationg , bactericidal protein-containing substances which are produced by certain strains of bacteria and are active against some other strains of the same or closely related species.
41. Bacteriosins are useful in the control of diseases. Bacteriocins produced by avirulent isolates are exploited to control diseases caused by virulent isolates of the same bacterium.

Reproduction of Bacteria

1. **Fission**
   - The most common mode of reproduction in bacteria.
   - The bacterial cells divide into two daughter cells.
   - It is asexual reproduction.
2. **Conjugation**
   - Genetic material of one cell is transferred to another cell during conjugation.
   - The two cells are genetically different.
   - The donor cell transfers part of its genome to the recipient cell.
   - Conjugation is one type of genetic recombination.
   - Genetic recombination refers to any process leading to the formation of a new individual which derives some of its gene from one parent and some from another, genetically different, parent.
3. **Transforamtion**
   - DNA from one type of bacterium is incorporated into the genetic makcup of another organism during transformation.
   - In this DNA is absorbed through external source,This is amethod employed in laboratory to bring about recombination : but it may be occurring in nature as well.
4. **Transduction**
   - Virus that infects bacteria is called bacteriophage.
   - Bacteriophage grows within a bacterial cell.
   - The infected bacterial cell bursts and the bacteriophage particles are liberated.
   - Some of the bacteriophage particles released carry some genetic material of the host bacterial cell.
   - They enter into another bacterial cell and the genetic material brought into the cell by the virus is incorporated into that of the bacteria .
   - By this process a new genotype of the bacterium arises and this process is called transduction.

Gram Staining

- Gram staining is useful to distinguish plant pathogens.
- Based on gram stain reaction, the bacteria can be grouped as gram positive and gram negative.

- To do the gram staining the bacterial smear is prepared and subjected to the following solutions in the order listed: crystal violet, iodine solution, alcohol, and saffranin.
- Gram positive bacteria retain the crystal violet and hence appear deep violet in color.
- Gram negative bacteria lose the crystal violet and counterstained by the saffranin, and hence appear red in color.
- Gram negative bacterial cell walls contain minor of lipids. Alcohol treatment extracts the lipid and the crystal violet-iodine complex is also extracted.
- The crystal violet-iodine complex is retained in gram positive bacteria during alcohol treatment.
- Most of the plant pathogenic bacteria is gram negative.

Gram positive vs Gram negative bacteria

Sl.No	Gram Positive bacteria	Gram Negative bacteria
1.	Cell wall is thicker and homogemous	Cell wall is thinner and usually thin layered.
2.	Contains lower content of lipids (5-10%)	Contains higher content of lipids (up to 40%)
3.	Peptidoglycan comprises up to 90% of the cell wall and hence maximum lipid	Peptidoglycan comprises only 10%.
4.	Techoic acid present	Techoic acid absent
5.	Cell wall has higher amino sugar content (10-20%)	Low content of amino sugars
6.	Cell wall is simple in shape and is single layered.	Varying cell wall shape and is tripartite (3-layered).
7.	Mesosomes more prominent.	Mesosomes less prominent.
8.	Retains violet dye	Retains red dye
9.	Examples: Bacillus, Clavibacter, Streptomyces	Examples: Erwinia, Pseudomonas, Xanthomonas, Agrobacterium, Xylella

General Characters of Plant Pathogenic Bacteria

1. Barring Streptomyces, which is filamentous, Almost all plant pathogenic bacteria are rod shaped.
2. The rod shaped bacteria are more or less short and cylindrical and in young cultures, they range from 0.6 to 3.5 m in length and from 0.5 to 1.0 m in diameter.
3. Sometimes deviations from the rod shape in the form of a club, a Y or V shaped, and other branched forms occur, and some bacteria may occasionally occur in pairs or in short chains.

4. The cell walls of bacteria of most species are enveloped by a viscous, gummy material, which may be thin (Slime layer) or may be thick, forming a relatively large mass around the cell (Capsule).
5. Most plant pathogenic bacteria are equipped with delicate, thread like flagella.
6. In some bacterial species each bacterium has only the flagellum, others , have a tuff of flagella at one end of the cell Polar flagella some have a single flagellum or a tuft of flagella at each end, and till others have peritrichous flagella, that is, distributed over the entire surface of the cell.
7. In the filamentous Streptomyces species, the cells consist of non septate branched threads, which usually have a spiral formation and produce conidia in chains on aerial hyphae.
8. Single bacterium appears hyaline or yellowish white under the compound microscope.
9. Bacteria grow and produce colonies on solid medium.
10. Colonies of different species may vary in size, shape, form of edges, elevation and colour, and are sometimes characteristics of a given species.
11. Bacterial cells have thin, relatively tough, and somewhat rigid cell walls.
12. All the material inside the cell wall constitutes the protoplast.
13. The nuclear material consist of a large circular chromosome composed DNA and appear as spherical, ellipsoidal or dumbbell shaped body within the cytoplasm.
14. Often bacteria also have single or multiple copies of addition smaller circular chromosomes called ‘Plasmids’ that can move or be moved between bacteria or between bacteria and plants as for example in the crown gall disease.
15. Rod shaped Phytopathogenic bacteria reproduce by the asexual process known as binary fission or fission. Under favourable conditions bacteria may divide every 20 minutes.
16. Almost all plant pathogenic bacteria develop mostly in the host plant as parasites and partly in plant debris or in the soil as saprophytes.

Important Plant Pathogenic Bacteria

Morphology

It is the study of size, shape, structure, and arrangement of cells.

(a) Size of Bacteria

Bacteria are very small or minute, as single drop of water may contains about 50 billions of bacteria are usually measured in micrometer (μm) which is equivalent to 1/1000 mm.

1. Size may varies depending upon the species. Size generally ranges from 1 to 10 microns.
2. Most of the bacterial cells 0.5 to 1 μm in width or diameter.
3. Cylindrical or rod (Baclli) 2-3 μm length.
4. Spiral or helical (Spirlli) – 0.75 -1.25 μm.

b) Shape in Bacteria:

The shapes of bacterial cells are

1. Spherical or Ellipsoidal or Oval – Cocci
2. Cylindrical or rod- Bacilli
3. Spiral or Helical – Spirilli

Some species have variety of shapes and thus termed as pleomorphic. e.g. Arthrobacter.

c) Arrangement of Bacterial Cells

Bacterial cells are arranged in a characteristic manner of the particular species. The typical pattern of cell arrangement in different bacteria is an important characteristics used in identification of bacteria.

d) Cell grouping or Arrangement in Cocci:

i) **Monococcus:** Single spherical bacterial cell.

ii) **Diplococcus:** A coccus divides into two plane and cells remains in pairs.

iii) **Streptococcus:** A coccus is arranged in a long chain e.g. *Streptococcus* sp.

iv) **Tetrad:** A coccus divides in two plans, second division at a right angle to the first plane of division and forms a square of four cells. e.g. *Tetracoccus* sp.

v) **Sarcina:** A cube of eight coccus cell is formed by three divisions in alternate planes at right angle to each other. A cube of eight cells is known as Sarcina.

vi) **Staphylococci:** A coccus cells divides in three planes in irregular pattern like cluster of cells or bunch of grapes. E.g. *Staphylococcus albus*

vii) **Vibrio:** The short comma shaped cells are called as Vibrio. Short tightly coined rods are called spirillum. Vey long cell with several cuvves and twiste are called “Spirochete”.

e) Cell Grouping or Arrangement in Bacilli:

i) **Monobacilli:** Single rod shaped bacterial cell. e.g. *Monobacillus.*

ii) **Diplobacilli:** Bacilli are arranged in a pair of two cells. e.g. *Bacillus subtilis.*

iii) **Streptobacilli:** Cells are arranged in a chain. e.g. *Lactobacillus bukgaricus.*

iv) **Palisade:** Group of cells lined side by side like matchsticks in a match box called as palisade arrangement.

f) Flagellar Arrangement in Bacteria:

All types of bacteria do not have a flagella they are mostly present in *bacilli* and *spirilli* and rarely in cocci.

i) **Atrichous:** A cell without flagella.

ii) **Monotrichous:** Single polar flagellum at one end.

iii) **Amphitrichous:** A cell with a single polar flagellum at both the ends. E.g Spirillim.

iv) **Lophotrichous:** A cell having tuft or bunch of flagella at both the ends. E.g. Coli.

v) **Cephalotrichous:** A cell having a pair of flagella at both end.

g) Arrangement in Spirilli:

The spirilli are predominantly unattached however they differ in frequency of turns and overall length. They are grouped in three types as:

(a) Short tightly coiled rod called spirillum.

b) Short incomplete spirals called as comma or vibrios.

c) They are long twisted with several curves calls "Spirochete".

Classification of Plant Pathogenic Bacteria

The bacteria belongs to the clas Schizomycetes. Plant pathogenic belongs to 3 different orders .

1. Order: Pseudomonadales

Family: Pseudomonadaceae

Important Characters

- It does not produe non water soluble pigment.
- It produces soluble pigment which is not yellow.
- No acid is produced from lactose.

Genera: ***Pseudomonas***

Important Characters

- It does not produce non water soluble pigment.
- It produces soluble pigment which is not yellow.
- No acid is produced from lactose.

Important Plant Pathogens

Sl. No	Name of Pathogen	Name of disease
1	*Pseudomonas solanacearum*	Wilts of Tomato, Banana, Brinjal, Potato
2	*Pseudomonas tabaci*	Wild fire of tobacco
3	*Pseudomonas syringae* pv. *phaseolicola*	Halo blight of beans

Genera: *Xanthomonas*

Important Characters

- Culture develop an yellow non water soluble pigment.
- Produce acid from lactose.

Important Plant Pathogens

Sl.No	Name of Pathogen	Name of disease
1	*Xanthomons campestris*	Black rot of cabbage
2	*Xanthomons campestris* pv. *oryzae*	Bacterial blight of rice
3	*Xanthomons campestris pv. citri*	Citrus canker
	Xanthomons campestrispv. malvacearum	Black arm of cotton

2. Order: Eubacteriales

I. Family: Enterobacteriaceae

Important Characters

- The bacterial cells are gram negative and motile with peritrichous flagella.
- They produce acid from sugars.

Genus: *Erwinia*

Important Plant Pathogens

Sl. No	Name of Pathogen	Name of disease
1	*Erwinia amylovora*	Fire blight of apple
2	*Erwinia carotovora*	Soft rot of many vegetables

II. Family: Rhizobeaceae

Important Characters

- The cells are rod shaped, gram negative and sparsely flagellated.
- The colonies are white.
- The genus *Agrobacterium* is pathogenic on plants.

Genus: *Agrobacterium*

Important Plant Pathogens

Sl.No	Name of Pathogen	Name of disease
1	*Agrobacterium tumefaciens*	Crown gall in many cells

III. Family: Corynebacteriaceae

Important Characters

- The bacterial cells are gram positive.
- *Corynebacterium* is the only gram positive plant pathogen while others are gram negative.
- The bacterial cells are pleomorphic rod that show the characteristic arrangement produced by snapping division.
- They are motile rods.

Genus: Corynebacterium

Important Plant Pathogens

Sl.No	Name of Pathogen	Name of disease
1.	*Corynebacterium michiganense*	Bacterial wilt of tomato
2.	*Corynebacterium tritici*	Tundu disease of wheat
3.	*Corynebacterium sepedonicum*	Leaf spot and wilt in many crops
4.	*Corynebacterium insidiosum*	Leaf spot of many crops
5.	*Corynebacterium rathayi*	Gummosis in many crops

3. Order: Actinomycetales

Family: Streptomycetaceae

Important Characters

- It produces conidia in aerial hyphae in chains.
- It has characteristic branching mycelium and spores are formed by fragmentation of the plasma straight or rod shaped .

Important Plant Pathogens

Sl.No	Name of Pathogen	Name of disease
1	*Streptomyces scabies*	Potato scab

Mode of Entry

Bacteria cannot penetrate host tissues as they do not have germ tubes and appresorium. They enter the host through different types of natural opening.

S. No.	Pathogen	Enter through	Disease
1	*Streptomyces scabies*	Lenticels	Scab of potato
	Pseudomonas tabaci	Stomata	Wild fire of tobacco
2	*Xanthomonas phaseoli*	Stomata	Bean blight
	Xanthomonas campestris	Stomata	Black rot of cabbage
	Xanthomonas campestris pv. malvacearum	Stomata	Angular leaf spot of cotton.
3	*Xanthomonas campestris pv. oryzae*	Wounds	Bacterial blight of rice
	Erwinia spp.	Wounds	Soft rot of vegetables
	Agrobacterium tumefaciens	Wounds	Crown gall of fruit trees
4	*Xanthomonas campestris*	Hydathodes	Black rot of cabbage
5	*Erwinia amylovora*	Floral parts	Fire blight of apple

Mode of Spread

S. No.	Transmitted through	Pathogen	Disease
1	Seed	*Xanthomonas malvacearum* *Xanthomonas campestris pv. oryzae*	Black arm of cotton Bacterial blight of rice
2	Soil	*Pseudomonas solanacearum*, *Xanthomonas campestris pv. malvacearum*	Wilts of Tomato, Banana, Brinjal, Potato, Cotton
3	Insect		
I	Honey bees	*Erwinia amylovora*	Fire blight of apple
II	Corn flea beetle	*Xanthomonas stewartii*	Corn wilt
4	Nemaode		
I	*Anguina tritici*	*Corynbacterium tritici*	Tundu disease of wheat
II	*Meloidogyne var. acrita*	*Pseudomonas solanacearum*	Wilt of tomato
5	Crop debris	*Xanthomonas malvacearum*	Black arm of cotton

Perpetuation of Bacteria

The phytopathogenic bacteria do not produce any resting structures. They survive by some of the following ways:

1. Survival on Self Sown Plant, Collateral Hosts

Bacterial pathogen survives and multiplies on self sown plants of host crop, collateral hosts during the main and the off seasons. The collateral hosts are most often perennial or noxious weeds growing in the host crop fields, or in their vicinity while others may be cultivated economic crop plants. The host range of some bacterial plant pathogens is very wide.

e. g *Pseudomonas solaneceanum* -200 host plants.

Agrobacterium tumefaciens- 150 host plants.

2. Survival on Host Crop

The pathogens of the bacterial leaf blight and the leaf streak of rice may survive from crop to crop in double or triple – rice culture areas in the tropics. The latent infections as in cankers, galls, bud scales, the cracks in the bark or sheltered place are often further protected by the host mucilage in trees as in the citrus canker or the fire blight.

3. Survival on Non Host Plants

Xanthomonas campestris pv. citri causal agent of citrus canker has been found to survive in the non-host plants. The epiphytic (Saprophytic) existence of *X.campestris pv. phasebli* on the phyllosphere of *Phaseolus vulgaris* has been found.

4. Survival through Crop Residues and in Soil

Some of the Phytopathogenic bacteria are capable of living saprophytically on plant residues or parennate in the soil in free state or on any organic matter. e.g *Erwinia* spp. *Pseudomonas, solanacearum racee2, Xanthomoans campestris pv. malvacearum*. Most of the bacterial pathogens of aerial parts can not survive in a natural soil for a long time due to their poor competitive saprophytic ability and antagonism of other microorganisms.

5. Survival through Seeds and Vegetative Propagation Parts

Some of the phyopathogenic bacteria survive in seeds of some crops and vegetative plant parts used for propagation e. g *Xanthomonas campestris pv. oyzae* and *Xanthomonas compestris pv. malvacearum* survive through seeds. *Pseudomonas solanacearum* survive in potato tubers.

Important Phytopathogenic Bacteria

S.. No	Genus	Gram Reaction	Characters	Symptoms produced on host	Example
1	*Pseudomonas*	Gram-ve	1. Rod straight to curved, size 0.5-1 X 1.5-4 μ m, one to many polar flagella. 2.Colonies not yellow, do not produce acid from lactose.	Leaf spot, blights, vascular wilts, soft rots, canker.	1. Brown rot or bacterial wilt of potato. 2 Bacterial wilt of brinjal and tomato.

2	*Xanthomonas*	Gram-ve	1. Straight rods, size 0.4-1X 1.2 -3 μ m. One polar flagellum present. 2. Colonies yellow due to Xanthomonadin, produce acid from lactose.	Leaf spot, fruit spots, blight, canker	1. Citrus canker, 2. Black arm of cotton, 3.Blight of paddy.
4	*Erwinia*	Gram-ve	1. Straight rods, size 0.5-1, 0-3.0 μ m , several peritrichous flagella.	Fire blight, wilt, soft rot.	1. Fire blight of apple. 2. Soft rot of vegetables.
5	*Clavibactor (Corynebacterium)*	Gram-ve	Straight to straightly curved rods, 0.5-0.9X 1.5 -4.0 μ m. non motile but some species are motile by one or two polar flagella.	Wilt	Wilt of potato ad Tomato
6	*Streptomyces*	Gram-ve	Slender branched hyphae without cross walls 0.5-2 μ m diameter.	Scab	Potato scab

Management of Bacterial Diseases

Bacterial plant pathogens directly enter the host tissue either through natural openings or through wounds; therefore, it is tricky to manage them. Some of the general principles of managing the bacterial disease are as follows:

1. Plant Sanitation

These measures are adopted so as to avoid the disease onset and also to prevent spread. e.g.

i) Collection and destruction of diseased fallen leaves, bolls etc. for bacterial blight of cotton.

ii) Removal of dead plant parts from fruit crops and protection of cut surface with suitable bactericides (e. g for citrus canker and fire blight of apple).

ii) Avoiding injuries to the plant parts at the time of cultural operations and during harvest, transport and storage.

2. Exclusion

Exclusion of a disease entry either from a foreign nation or within the country, from a diseased to a healthy tract is an effective measure for avoiding the disease. Quarantine measures are in vogue in several countries. e .g diseased managed: Citrus canker.

3. Eradication

Eradication is generally carried out for eliminating a well established pathogen and its host plant, collateral hosts, or insect vectors and some times use of cultural measures for starving out or killing the pathogen.

i) Pruning of the infected twigs is followed to reduce the inoculums in orchards for citrus canker.

ii) The destruction of volunteer plants and weed hosts brings down the inoculum level. e.g Brown rot of potato .

iii) The crop residue may be burnt or ploughed deep into the soil with watering to ensure decomposition, which is helpful for the pathogens which cannot live saprophytically in the soil. e. g. Bacterial blight of cotton .

iv). Crop rotation with cereals is advocated for the management of wilt of tobacco.

v) The balanced application of NPK , particularly low and split doses of N, helps to reduce the intensity of the bacterial leaf blight of rice.

vi) The control of vectors is helpful in reducing the citrus canker and soft rot of vegetables (*Erwinia* spp.) .

vii) The avoidance of cultural mismanagement favourable to disease is important viz., flooding or over irrigation in the field (against the soft rot disease) and water logging in the nurseries (against the bacterial leaf blight of rice).

ix) The sterilization of the cutting knife by flame or by 0.1 % KMNO4 solution while cutting the potato tuber for sowing is recommended against the potato wilt.

x) The seed certification programes to raise pathogen free seeds.

xi) Elimination of the externally and internally seed born pathogen by seed treatment. e.g.

1. Soaking of rice seeds in 0.025% strpetocyclic solution for leaf blight disease of rice.
2. Delinting of cotton seed with concentrated sulphuric acid for bacterial blight of cotton.
3. Hot water treatment of cotton seed at 56^0 C for 10 minutes for bacterial blight of cotton.

xii) When tobacco is immediately grown after maize there is a considerable reduction in the incidence of *Pseudomonas solanacearum* on the later host.

4. Plant Protection

Plant Protection measures are adopted to prevent the commencement and subsequent spread of plant diseases. e. g

i) Seed treatment of rice and cotton with antibiotics against bacterial blight and leaf streak diseases respectively.

ii) Treatment of seed tubers of potato with stroptocycline @ 0.02% for 30 minutes, against brown rot disease.

iii) Foliar sprays with Bordeaux mixture and copper oxychloride against leaf spots and blights.

iv) Foliar sprays of streptomycin sulphate, 100 and 500 ppm against citrus canker and fire blight of apple.

v) Therapy: Pancillin and vancomycin are effective in the disintegration of the crow gall. The application of antibiotics for protection also involves therapy. The bacteriocines have also been demonstrated to be successful against bacterial disease e. g *Agrobacterium radiobacter* against crown gall of peach and tomato seedlings (*Agrobacterium fumetaciens.*)

vi) Immunization: By screening under artificial epiphytic conditions, resistance source for bacterial pathogens can be known. Resistant varieties are evolved by selection, breeding and other methods.

Prokaryotes: Classification of Prokaryotes according to Bergey's Manual of Systematic Bacteriology

Prokaryotes

Prokaryotic organisms are that in which nucleus is primitive type and nuclear material is not enclosed within the nuclear membrane.

Bacteria are placed in the kingdom "Prokaryotae" because of the prokaryotic cellular organization of the members. However, extremely diverse groups of microorganisms differing in morphological, physiological and ecological properties are found within this kingdom. In the beginning, description and information of bacterial systematics or classification was being published in the comprehensive volumes of "Bergey's Manual of Determinative Bacteriology" (1923, first edition). The 9th edition of Bergey's Manual, published in 1984 was the last of such comprehensive manual and from 1984 onwards it was renamed as "Bergey's *Manual of Systematic Bacteriology"*. It is the most widely accepted and used reference document or book for classification and identification of bacteria. In the 9th edition, the kingdom Prokaryota ((Monera) is divided into 4 divisons based on nature of the cell wall.These are: ***Graciliculte*s**; ***Firmicutes***; ***Tenericutes*** and ***Mendosicutes*** .

Kingdom: Prokaryota

Divisison 1. Gracilicutes

Important character

1. Usually gram reaction is negative.
2. Cell wall consisting of an outer membrane, a peptidoglycan layer and a unit membrane with fatty acid glycerol ester type lipid.
3. Endospore is not formed.
4. Divided into two classes- Proteobacteria and Oxyphotobacteria on the basis of phylogenetic principles.
5. All gram –ve plant pathogenic bacteria are included in proteobaceria and scattered in three main classes.

Divison 2. Firmicutes

Important character

1. Gram reaction is generally, but not always positive.
2. Cell wall consisting of a thick peptidoglycan and unit membrane but without an outer membrane.
3. Some produce endospores.
4. Divided into two classes of firmibacteria and thallobacteria
5. Bacillus and clostridium are included into Firmibacteria.
6. Actinomycetes and related bacteria such *as Streptomyces, Clavibacer, Rhodococcus*, *Curobacterium*, and *Nocardia* are included in Thallobacteria.

Divison 3. Tenericutes

Important character

- Prokaryotes that lack a cell wall.
- Highly polymorphic.
- The cells are enclosed by a unit membrane.
- Includes class Mollicutes in which plant pathogenic MLO (Phytoplasma and Spiroplasma) belong.

Divison 4. Mendosicutes

Important character

- The prokaryotes which have a cell envelop without conventional peptidoglycan or cell wall material are included.

- Cell walls are made entirely of heteropolysaccharides and protein macromolecules.
- Gram reaction is positive or negative.
- This divison has a single class- Archaeobacteria
- No plant pathogenic prokaryotes belongs to this divison.

The four divison are further divided into folling classes, orders and families;

Divison I	**Gracilicutes**	**Gram negative bacteria**
Class	Scotobacteria	Gram negative, non photosynthetic,bacteria
Class	Anoxyphotobacteria	Gram negative, photosynthetic bacteria that produce oxygen
Class	Oxyphotobacteria	Gram negative, photosynthetic bacteria that produce oxygen
Some families and genera under division Gracilicutes		
Family	**Genus**	
Neisseriaceae	Neisseria, Acinetobacter	
Pseudomonadaceae	Pseudomonas, Xanthomonas	
Azotobacteriaceae	Azotobacter	
Rhizobeaceae	Rhizobium, Agrobacterium	
Enterobacteriaceae	Erwinia, Enterobactor	
Vibrionaceae	Vibrio	
Bacterioidaceae	Bacterioids	
Spirochaetaceae	Spirochaeta	
Rickettsiaceae	Rickettsia	
Bartonellaceae	Bartonella	
Chlamydaceae	Chlamydia	
Divison II--	***Firmicutes***	**Gram positive bacteria**
Class	Firmibacteria	Gram positive rods and cocci
Class	Thallobacteria	Gram positive branching cells- the actinomycetes
Some families and genera under divison Firmicutes		
Family	**Genus**	
Microccaceae	Micrococus	
Peptococcaceae	Peptococcus	
Bacillaceae	Bacillus, Clostridium	
Lactobacaillaceae	Lactobacallus	
Propionibacteriaceae	Propiniobacterum	
Corynebacteriaceae	Corynebacterium	
Mycobacteraiceae	Mycobacterium	
Nocardiaceae	Nocardia	

Actinomycetaceae	Actinomycetes	
Streptomycetaceae	Streptomyces	
Streptococcaceae	Streptococcus	
Divison III	Tenericutes	Bacteria with soft or no cell walls
Class	Mollicutes	The Mycoplasmas
Some families and genera under divison Tenericutes		
Family	**Genus**	
Mycoplasmataceae	Mycoplasma, Ureaplasma	
Acholeplasmataceae	Acholeplasma	
Spiroplasmataceaee	Sprioplasma	
Divison IV	**Mendosicutes**	Bacteria that lack peptidoglycan in their cell wall
Class	Archaebacteria	Bacteria with typical compounds in the cell wall and the membranes

Model Question Papers

A. Objective Types

a. Multiple Choice Questions

1. In the classification of bacteria according to shape, which among the following refers to cuboidal arrangement of bacterial cells?
   (a) Tetrads (b) Staphylococci
   (c) Sarcinae (d) Streptococci

2. Ribosomes of prokaryotes have a sedimentation coefficient of?
   (a) 90S (b) 80S
   (c) 50S (d) 70S

3. The bacterial cells are gram negative and motile with peritrichous flagella.
   (a) Erwinia (b) Agrobacterium
   (c) Pseudomonas (d) Xanthomonas

4. Mobile DNA called
   (a) Plasmids (b) Episomes
   (c) Transposons (d) Karyosomes

5. Growth of bacteria or microorganisms refer to ________________
   (a) An increase in the size of an individual organism
   (b) An increase in the mass of an individual organism
   (c) Changes in the total population
   (d) An increase in number of cells

6. The first demonstration of recombination in bacteria was achieved by __________
   (a) Lederberg and Tatum (b) Luria and Delbruck
   (c) Joshua and Lederberg (d) Luria and Tatum
7. Peptidoglycan layer is present in large quantity in?
   (a) Gram-positive bacteria (b) Gram-negative bacteria
   (c) Fungi (d) Algae
8. Peptidoglycan is made up of __________
   (a) N-acetylglucosamine
   (b) N-acetylmuramic acid
   (c) N-acetylglucosamine, N-acetylmuramic acid
   (d) N-acetylglucosamine, N-acetylmuramic acid, amino acids
9. Teichoic acid present in Gram-positive bacteria can bind to which ion?
   (a) Fe ions (b) Phosphorus ions
   (c) Mg ions (d) Sulphur ions
10. Usually Gram negative bacteria belongs to division
    (a) Gracilicutes (b) Firmicutes
    (c) Tenericutes (d) Mendosicutes
11. Gram-negative bacteria are more resistant to antibiotics due to the presence of?
    (a) Thin peptidoglycan wall (b) Outer lipopolysaccharide layer
    (c) Porin proteins (d) Teichoic acid
12. Bacteria with less than a complete twist or comma shaped is known as?
    (a) Spirilla (b) Helical
    (c) Vibrio (d) Spirochetes
13. Usually Gram positive bacteria belongs to division
    (a) Gracilicutes (b) Firmicutes
    (c) Tenericutes (d) Mendosicutes
14. The bacterial cells with a single polar flagellum at both the ends.
    (a) Monotrichous (b) Lophotrichous
    (c) Peritrichous (d) Atrichous
15. Extra chromosomal DNA capable of autonomous replication
    (a) Plasmids (b) Episomes
    (c) Transposons (d) Karyosomes

16. Low molecular weight iron (III) transport agents
    (a) Siderophore (b) Episomes
    (c) Transposons (d) Karyosomes
17. Bacterial cell lacking cell wall is called
    (a) Protoplast (b) Spheroplast
    (c) Transposons (d) Karyosomes
18. The short comma shaped cells are called
    (a) Vibrio (b) Coccus
    (c) Sarcina (d) Tetrad
19. The colonies of which bacteria are white.
    (a) Erwinia (b) Agrobacterium
    (c) Pseudomonas (d) Xanthomonas
20. The bacteria which produce acid from lactose.
    (a) Erwinia (b) Agrobacterium
    c) Pseudomonas (d) Xanthomonas

Answer

Q. No	Answer	Q. No	Answer
1	(c) Sarcinae	11	(b) Outer lipopolysaccharide layer
2	(c) 70S	12	(c) Vibrio
3	(a) Erwinia	13	(b) Firmicutes
4	(c) Transposons	14	(b) Lophotrichous
5	(d) An increase in number of cells	15	(a) Plasmids
6	(a) Lederberg and Tatum	16	(a) Siderophore
7	(a) Gram-positive bacteria	17	(a) Protoplast
8	(d) N-acetylglucosamine, N-acetylmuramic acid, amino acids	18	(a) Vibrio
9	(c) Mg ions	19	(b) Agrobacterium
10	(a) Gracilicutes	20	(d) Xanthomonas

b. True/False

1. Most of the plant pathogenic bacteria are rod shaped .
2. Erwinia is anaerobic plant pathogenic bacteria .
3. Most of the plant pathogenic bacteria reproduce by asexual process known as binary fission.
4. Streptomyces are gram negative in Gram's reaction.

5. Bacillus species produce endosproes which are dormant structures.
6. Bacterial cell lacking cell wall is called protoplast.
7. The short comma shaped cells of bacteria are called as Vibrio.
8. The bacteria Pseudomonas produces soluble pigment which is not yellow.
9. The bacteria Xanthomonas donot produce acid from lactose.
10. Erwinia is gram negative bacteria having motile with peritrichous flagella.
11. Bacterial species are often distinguished from one another by Gram staining.
12. Fission is the most common mode of reproduction in bacteria.
13. Conjugation is one type of genetic recombination in bacteria.
14. Transforamtion is a method employed in laboratory to bring about recombination in bacteria.
15. *Streptomyces scabies* produces conidia in aerial hyphae in chains.

Answer

Question. No	Answer	Question No	Answer
1	True	9	True
2	True	10	True
3	True	11	True
4	False	12	True
5	False	13	True
6	True	14	True
7	True	15	True
8	True		

B. Descriptive Questions

a. Short snswer type questions

1. Which bacterial species and pathovars make up the greatest number of plant-pathogenic bacteria.
2. Which disease is recognized as having been the first to prove that bacteria are phytopathogenic.
3. List the top five genera of phytopathogenic bacteria.
4. What aspects of the environment are more likely to cause citrus canker disease?
5. Why are the biotechnologists spending so much time studying the organism that causes crown gall disease? .

6. List at least two other names for wheat tundu disease.
7. What bacteria is frequently linked to wheat tundu disease?
8. Which pathogenic races or strains of Pseudomonas solanacearum, the causative agent of solanaceous plant wilt, have been isolated from infected hosts in India?

b. Long answer

1. Write notes on the following plant pathogenic bacteria.

(i)	Pseudomonas	(ii)	Xanthomonas
(ii)	Agrobacterium	(iv)	Streptomyces

2. Give brief account of the following.

(i)	Reproduction in bacteria	(iii)	Causal organism of tundu disease of wheat

3. Describe the survival mechanisms of bacterial plant pathogens.
4. Describe the dispersal mechanisms of plant pathogenic bacteria.
5. Explain about horizontal gene transfer in bacteria.
6. Describe occurrence and importance, symptoms, causal organism, disease cycle, predisposing factors, and managment of any one of the following diseases.
   i. Citrus canker
   ii. Bacterial wilt of solanaceous plants.
7. What are the key characteristics that distinguish plant pathogenic bacteria from other bacteria, and how do these characteristics contribute to their pathogenicity?
8. Describe the role of bacterial biofilms in plant pathogenesis. How do biofilms contribute to the survival and persistence of plant pathogenic bacteria on plant surfaces and within plant tissues?
9. What are the major types of diseases caused by plant pathogenic bacteria, and how do these diseases impact agricultural production? Provide examples of specific bacterial diseases affecting crops.
10. Describe the role of environmental factors such as temperature, humidity, and soil composition in the development and spread of plant bacterial diseases. How do these factors influence the life cycle of bacterial pathogens?
11. Discuss the principles of integrated disease management (IDM) in controlling bacterial diseases in plants. How can cultural practices,

biological control agents, and chemical treatments be combined to effectively manage bacterial plant pathogens?

Other plant pathogens: Mollicutes; Flagellant protozoa; FVB; Green algae and parasitic higher plants

Mollicutes

- The Mollicutes are a class of bacteria distinguished by the *absence of a cell wall.*
- The word Mollicutes is derived from the Latin *mollis* (meaning *soft or pliable*) and *cutis* (meaning skin).
- They are parasites of various animals and plants, living on or in the hosts cells.
- Individuals are very small , typically only 0.2-0.3 μm in size and have a very small genome size.
- They vary in form, although most have sterols that make the cell membranes somewhat more rigid.
- Many are able to move about through *gliding*, but members of the genus *Spiroplasma* are helical and move by *twisting* .
- The best known genus in Mollicutes is *Mycoplasma.*

Phytoplasmas or Mycoplasma

Definition

Phytoplasmas are unicellular, ultramicroscopic, walless, prokaryotic, self-replicating, highly pleomorphic, filterable organisms or entities.

Mycoplasma lack rigid cell wall, being surrounded only by single triple unit membrane which allows them to be highly plemorphic. They assume vast array of shapes and size. They require sterols (Lipoproteins) for growth. Mycoplasma cannot be grown on artificial media and they reproduce by budding and binary fissions.

Taxonomic Position

Kingdom	Prokaryotic
Division	Firmicutes
Class	Mollicutes
Order	Acholeplasmatales
Family	Acholeplasmataceae
Genus	Candidatus Phytoplasma

Historical Background

1. Plant disease caused by MLO's were known since 1603 in Japan in Mulbery (Mulbery dwarf disease).
2. Mycoplasma –like organism or MLOs were first discovered by Doi *et al.,* in 1967.
3. MLO that infects plants have been reclassified as Phytoplasmas by Sears and Krikpatrick in 1994.
4. In 2004, the genus name of Phytoplasma was adopted and is currently at *Candidatus status* which is used for bacteria that cannot be cultured.

General Characters

1. They are wall less, surrounded by a unit membrane, and consist of cytoplasma, ribosomes and nuclear material.
2. Pleomorphic or filamentous shape with varying size ranging from 200 to 800 nm and is less than 1 μm in diameter.
3. DNA is present in cytoplasm. Genome is very small (689-1600kb).
4. They are very small and ultramicroscopic.
5. Strictly host dependent and can survive and multiply only in the sap of phloem sieve tubes or insect haemolymph; also in their eggs.
6. Only phloem –feeding insect vectors (Leafhoppers, Plant hoppers and Psllids) that possess piercing/sucking type mouth parts (Hemiptera) can potentially acquire and transmit the phytoplasma in a persistent propagative manner.
7. They cannot be grown on artificial media but can grow in alimentary canal, hemolymph, salivery glands, and interellularly in different body organisms of their insect vectors.
8. Reproduce by binary fission.
9. They are sensitive to tetracycline but resistant to penicillin.
10. MLOs have no flagella, produce no spore and are gram-ve.

Symptoms Produced by Phytoplasma in Plants

1. Phytoplasmas like bodies are now stated to be occur in more than 60 to 70 plant diseases, which are characterized by the growth abnormalities and yellowing of leaves.
2. Characteristic symptom of yellow type disease includes uniform yellowing or reddening of leaves, smaller leaves, shortening of internodes, stunting of plants and proliferation of auxiliary bud.

3. "Witch brooms" includes reduction of leaf size with leaves becoming brittle, excessive proliferation of shoots.
4. "Phyllody" replacement of floral parts of leaves greening or sterility of flowers and reduced yield. Finally more or less rapid dieback, decline and disorder after several years.
5. MLOs are mostly restricted to phloem tissue becomes; a phloem may provide favourable conditions for growth as phloem elements have a high osmotic pressure and slightly alkaline PH.

Disease caused by Phytoplasmas

(i) Pear decline
(ii) Grape yellows
(iii) Aster yellows of vegetables
(iv) Apple proliferation
(v) Little leaf of brinjal.
(vi) Coconut lethal yellowing
(vii) Elms yellows
(viii) Pigeonpea witche's broom
(ix) Rice yellow dwarf
(x) Stolbur
(xi) X.disease
(xii) Citrus greening
(xiii) Seasamum phyllody
(xiv) Grassy shoot of sugarcane
(xv) Little leaf of Brinjal

Management of Phytoplasmas

1. Most of the control measures against yellow type of disease are avoided at preventing infections.
2. Heat Treatment:Phytoplasmas are thermolabile and are destroyed or inactivated at or above 40 to 50^{0}C. It is possible to cure yellow infected plants grassy shoot of sugarcane by heat treatment.
3. Use of antibiotics: Antibiotics are known to suppress the yellow type disease. The most effective antibiotics appear to be chloro tetracycling, oxy tetra cycline and tetra cycline with choramphenicol or ledermycin. The application of antibiotics by root dip or paste under tha bark, standing cutting in solution appears to be more effective than foliar spray or soil drenches.

4. Vector Control: Since most of disease are spread by the vector, control of vector through effective insecticides like Thiomethoxam, Imidacloprid ,Rogar, Malathion.
5. Kiliing of alternate hosts: Weeds may serve as alternate host, hence killing of alternate host.

Spiroplasma

Definition

Spiro plasma is a wall less mollicutes bounded by a triple layered unit membrane.

Taxonomic Position

Kingdom	Prokaryotic
Division	Tenericutes
Class	Mollicutes
Order	Endoplasmatales
Family	Spiroplasmataceae
Genus	Spiroplasma

General Characters

1. They lack true cell wall ,bounded by a single triple layered unit membrane.
2. They produce typical 'fried egg' like colonies on agar medium.
3. They multiplied by fission.
4. They produce helical (100-240 nm in dia., 2-4µm inlength) form in liquid culture medium.
5. Can be cultured on nutrient media.
6. Resistant to penicillin but inhibited by tetracyeline.
7. Transmitted only through phloem –feeding insect vectors mostly through leaf hoppers.
8. Mostly found in the gut or haemolymph of insects, or in the phloem of infected plants.

Disease caused by Spiroplasma

(i) Corn stunt

(ii) White bud of maize

(iii) Cirtus stubborn

Management of Spiroplasma

1) Use of disease resistant planting stocks.
2) Eradication of infected trees in early stages of infection.
3 Vector Control: Since most of disease are spread by the vector, control of vector through effective insecticides like Rogar, Malathion, Endosulphan etc.

Fastidious Vascular Bacteria (Rickettesia Like Organisms)

General Characters

1. The fastidious vascular bacteria were formally known as rickettesia like organisms (RLOs).
2. They are usually rod shaped, aflagellate, bounded by a cell membrane and a cell wall measuring 1.0 -4.0x 0.2-0.5µm.
3. They are confined to phloem or xylem of the host plant but never to both.
4. Usually transmitted by leaf hoppers exception: Citrus greening bacteria (*Liberobacter asciaticum* is transmitted by citrus psylla (*Diaphorina citri*).
5. Al most all fastidious bacteria known so far are gram negative .Exception. Sugarcane ratoon stunting (*Clavibacter xyli pv.xyli*) is gram positive in nature.
6. There are two groups: one in which the fastidious bacteria occur only in phloem (phloem limited) and the other in which they occur in xylem (i.e xylem limited).
7. Xylem limited fastidious bacteria known so far have been successfully grown on nutrient media while phloem limited fastidious bacteria have not been culture so far.
8. They are sensitive to antibiotics such as tetracycline and penicillin and to high temperature.

Disease caused by Fastidious vascular bacteria

(i) Plecei's disease of grapes
(ii) Almond leaf scorch
(iii) Alfalfa dwarf
(iv) Phony peach
(v) Raton stunting
(vi) Plum leaf scald.

Management

1. Heat treatment of entire plant parts or propagative plant parts, by immersing them in water kept at 45-50^{0}C for 2-3 hours or by keeping the plants or plant propagules in hot air at 45 to 50^{0}C for 2-3 hours.It has been helpful in curing the sugarcane and grapevines from ratoon stunting disease and pierce's disease, respectively.
2. Use of antibiotics: Antibiotics are known to suppress fastidious vascular bacteria. The most effective antibiotics appear to be penicillin and tetracyclin.

Algae

General characters

1. Algae are the eukaryotic thallophytes having chlorophyll as their primary photosynthetic pigments. They are aerobic, photosynthetic organisms; contain three types of pigments chlorophyll, cartoenoids and phycocyanin.
2. They are ubiquitous organisms abundantly present in aquatic environment.
3. They have wide range of shapes and size and the common shapes are rhizoidal, filamentous and mucilaginous.
4. The Chlorophycean (green algae) cause disease in plants
5. Most of the algae are photoautotrophic, may reproduce either sexually or asexually.
6. Algae reproduce asexually by binary fission, fragmentation and formation of spores and sexually by formation of zygotes.
7. They spread through an air borne sporangia and produces 300 spores.
8. They entry in to the host through stomata and other natural openings.

Example

Red rust of tea, coffee, mango citrus, and guava (*Cephaleurous parasitica, Cephaleurous minimum, Cephaleurous coffeae)*

Management of Algae

1. Application of nitrogen and potassium significantly reduce the disease. Drainage should be provided.
2. All badly diseased or dead wood should be removed.
3. Pruning is recommended for tea, citrus, and cacao trees for the control of this disease.

4. Clsoe plucking of tea should be discouraged.
5. Irrigation reduces red rust due to an increase in host vigour.
6. Bordeaux mixture, copper oxychloride and cuprous oxide can be sprayed to control the disease.

Protozoa

General characters

1. Protozoa are single celled, non photothetic, eukaryotic animal like organisms. They are widely distributed in nature particularly in aquatic, environment or moist habitats.
2. Their size ranges from 2-3 micron.
3. They lack rigid cell wall and do not contain chlorophyll.
3. They make their movements with the help of cilia, flagella or pseudopodia.
4. Most of the protozoa are free living but some are symbiotic or parasitic causing diseases in plants animals and humans.
6. Free living protozoa are commonly found in fresh water salt water, sand, soil and decaying organic matter.
7. Protozoa reproduce sexually or asexually.
8. Asexual reproduction is either by binary fission or by budding or by both.
9. Sexual reproduction is by fusion of two gametes.
10. They have characteristics ability to regenerate the lost parts of the body. For example, Genera: Amoeba, Paramecium etc.

Example

1. Phloem necrosis of coffee (*Phytomonas leptovasorum*)
2. Hart rot of coconut and oil palm (Phytomonas)
3. Sudden wilt of oil palm
4. Empty root of Cassava

Prions

1. Resembling viruses that lacks nucleic acid (DNA or RN(a) and have infectious proteins molecule which were 100 times smaller than the smallest known virus, for which Prusiner coined the term prions, which comes from proteinaceous infectious particles that lack nucleic acid.
2. It is the smallest known protein aften considered to be the cause various infectious diseases of the nervous system.

3. Prions are some times called slow viruses because of their slow effect.
4. Prions are transmissible particles and cause mad cow disease, Creutzfeldt-Jakob disease in humans and Scrapie disease in sheep.
5. However, no plant diseases are reported to be caused by prions.

Nematodes

Introduction

1. Nematodes belong to the Animal kingdom, and phylum Nematoda.
2. The body of nematodes is elongate (thread like; nema in Greek means thread) without any segment.
3. It is cylindrical tapering at each end especially towards the tail.
4. Most of the important parasitic genera belong to the order Tylenchida and few under Dorylaimida.

General morphology

1. Plant parasitic nematodes mostly measure 300-1000 μm with some up to 4 mm long x 15-35 μm wide.
2. The body of the adult male is cylindrical, filiform, eel-shaped, made up of cuticle, hypodermis and somatic muscles, round in cross section and tapering at each end.
3. The anterior end is smooth, provided with papillae, leading to a buccal cavity and to oesophagus.
4. The body cavity between the gut and the body wall is usually regarded as a pseudocoelom containing a pseudocoelomic fluid.
5. Body is smooth, unsegmented without leg or other appendages.
6. The females of some species become swollen at adult stage and have pear-shapes (pyriform) or spheroid bodies.
7. Nematodes can be easily observed under microscope.
8. A valve is located at the junction of oesophagus and the intestine, the latter opening into the rectum and anus at the posterior end of the body.
9. The entire body is covered with a colourless, impermeable (permeable only to water) smooth or transversely striated cuticle with a sub-cuticular and muscular layer.

Nervous system

1. The nervous system consists of a nerve ring which encircles the gut usually in the region of the oesophageal isthmus.
2. Several nerves extend anteriorly and posteriorly.

Excertory system

1. A excretory duct opens at the exterior via an excretory pore.
2. The gut is an internal tube beginning at the oral opening and ending at the ventrally placed anus in juveniles and females and at the cloaca in male.

Reproductive system

1. Female have avulva in the mid body region with paired reproductive tracts.
2. The reproductive tract consists of an ovary, oviduct, uterus, vagina and vulva.
3. Male have single or paired tests, seminal vesicle and vasdeferens.
4. The vasdeferens opens into the cloaca which has a ventrally placed opening.
5. Males usually have a pair of copulatory spicules that lies in an invagination of the cloacal wall.
6. There are sclerotized structures such as a gubernaculums or lateral accessory pieces which guide the spicules.

Life cycle and reproduction of nematodes

1. The female lay eggs after copulation.
2. The young one from the egg is called larve.
3. The nematodes usually moult four times to reach the adult stage.
4. Appearance and structure of larvae are usually similar to the adults.
5. Larvae start to grow and each larval state is terminated by molt.
6. Nematodes usually moult four times to reach the adult stage.
7. Usually, first molt occurs in the egg and the final molt differentiates into adult male and female.
8. Fertile eggs are produced by females after mating with a male, or parthenogenetically in absence of males or can produce sperm herself.
9. A life cycle from egg to egg stage is completed with 3 to 4 weeks or requires slightly longer period in cooler temperature.

Behaviour of nematodes in soil

1. All plant parasitic nematodes, with the exception of free-living nematodes, complete a portion of their life cycle in soil.
2. Being soil-borne microfauna, the activities of these nematodes are affected by soil temperature, moisture, aeration, soil texture and pH,

organic matter, rhizosphere and various cultural operations. Population of nematodes is high in soil layer of 0-15 cm depth and sometimes they can live upto the depth of 150 cm or more.

3. Generally, concentration of nematodes is extremely high in the rhizosphere of susceptible host plants.
4. Movement of nematode in soil is very slow and a nematode can travel a maximum of one meter per season.
5. However, they can move faster at certain soil moisture level when pores are lined with thin film of water under water logging conditions.
6. In gall forming nematodes, temperature-moisture interaction determines the emergence of larvae from galls.
7. Most nematodes eggs hatch freely in water in absence of any special stimulus.
8. Nematodes are spread in a local areas by farm equipments, irrigation, flood or drainage water, animal feet and dust storms while spread to a longer distance through farm produce and nursery plants.

Signs and Symptoms

Typical root symptoms indicating nematode attack are root knots or galls, root lesions, excessive root branching, injured root tips, and stunted root systems. Symptoms on the above-ground plant parts indicating root infection are a slow decline of the entire plant, wilting even with ample soil moisture, foliage yellowing, and fewer and smaller leaves. These are, in fact, the symptoms that would appear in plants deprived of a properly functioning root system. Bulb and stem nematodes produce stem swellings and shortened internodes. Bud and leaf nematodes distort and kill bud and leaf tissue.

Examples of highly damaging plant parasitic nematodes

Tle plant parasitic nematodes belong to class: Nematodea; Subclass : Secernetia: Order: Tylenchida: Suborder: Tylenchina and Aphlenchina. A number of genera and species of nematodes are highly damaging to a great range of hosts, including foliage plants, agronomic and vegetable crops, fruit and nut trees, turfgrass, and forest trees. Some of the most damaging nematodes are:

1	Root knot	*Meloidogyne* spp
2	Cyst	*Heterodera* and *Globodera* spp
3	Root lesion	*Pratylenchus* spp.
4	Spiral	*Helicotylenchus* spp.
5	Burrowing	*Radopholus similis*

6	Bulb and stem	*Ditylenchus dipsaci*
7	Reniform	*Rotylenchulus reniformis*
8	Dagger	*Xiphinema* spp
9	Bud and leaf	*Aphelenchoides* spp

Nematodes as vector of plant pathogens

1. Some species of nematodes viz., dagger nematode (*Xiphinema* sp.), needle nematode (*Longidorus* spp. and *Paralongidorus* spp.) and stubby-root nematodes (*Trichodorus* spp. and *Paratrichodorus* spp.) can carry plant viruses.
2. Members of *Longidorus* and *Xiphinema* (family Longidoridae) transmit the polyhedral nepoviruses (type member : tobacco ringspot virus) while *Trichodours* and *Paratrichodorus* (family Trichodoridae) transmit the straight tubular tobraviruses (type member: tobacoo rattle virus).

Few examples of the nematodes as virus vectors are mentioned below:

Sl, No	Plant virus transmitted	Nematode species involved as vector
1	Arabis mosaic	*Longidorus caespiticola, Paralongidorus maximus, Xiphinema index,*
2	Brome mosaic	*Longidorus macrosoma, Xiphinema coxi, Xiphinema diversicaudatum*
3	Carnation ringspot	*Longidorus elongatus, Xiphinema diversicaudatum*
4	Cowpea mosaic	*Xiphinema basiri*
5	Grapevine fan leaf	*Xiphinema index* and *Xiphinema italiae*
6	Grapevine vein banding	*Xiphinema index*
7	Mulberry ringspot	*Longidorus martini*
8	Tobacco ringspot	*Xiphinema americanum, Xiphinema coxi*
9	Tomato ringspot	*Xiphinema americanum, Xiphinema brevicolle*
10	Tobacco rattle	*Paratrichodorus minor, Trichodorus cylindricus, Trichodorus primitives*

Plant parasitic nematode management

Nematode management should be multifaceted. Since eliminating nematodes is not possible, the goal is to manage their population, reducing their numbers below damaging levels. Common management methods used include

- Use of disease-resistant varieties
- Crop rotation
- Cultural practices
- Soil solarizarion
- Biological control

- Chemical control
- Quarantine
- Soil amendment

Phanerogamic Parasites

Fungi, nematodes, bacteria, and viruses are probably the first things that come to mind when thinking of plant pathogens. These organisms certainly do cause damage to plants of economic importance, but it may surprise you to know that parasitic flowering plants are also important pathogens.There are few seed plants, which are parasitic on living plants and are called parasitic higher plants or **Phanerogamic parasites.** These parasitic higher plants attack some valuable crops and trees causing considerable losses. They produce flowers and seeds and belongs to several widely separated botanical families they differ to each other on their dependency on host plants. These parasites have haustoria as absorbing organ, which sent deep into the vascular bundle of the host to draw water and nutrients. More than 2500 species of higher plants are known to live parasitically on other plants.

Classification of flowering plant parasites:

i) Complete Parasite (Holoparasites):

a. Root: Orobanchea (Broom rape)
b. Stem: Cuscuta (Dodder Amarvel)

ii) Partial Parasites (Semi Parasites)

a. Root: Striga (Sandle wood witch weed)
b. Stem: Loranthus (Banda or Deudrophae)

Complete Root Parasite - Broom Rape

Family: Orobanchaceae

Genus: Orobanche

1. Orobanche spp. are total root parasites affecting Tobacco, Brinjal, Tomato, Cauliflower, Turnip and many other solanaceous and cruciferous plants. . In some areas of the world, broom rape cause losses varying from 15 to 70 % of the crop.
2. The parasite consists of a stount, fleshy stem 15 to 50 cm long. This stem is yellow or brownish red in colour and is covered by small thin and brown scaly leaves.
3. The flower appearing in the axil of the leaves are white and tubular seeds are very small and black in colour and many remain viable in soil for several years.

4. The haustoria of the parasite penetrate into the root of the hosts and draw it nourishment.
5. When the host is carefully uprooted, the parasitic roots are seen intertwined with the host root systems; the growth of the host is retarded and remains stunted.

Management

1. Long crop rotation.
2. Destroy the parasite before flowering.
3. Drenching of the soil with 0.25% copper sulphate solution has been reported to be successful in destroying the parasites.
4. Fumigating the soil with methyl bromide.
5. Broom tapes is also effectively controled after treatment with the herbicides "Glyphosate".

Complete Stem Parasite - Dodder

Family: Cuscutaceae

Genus: Cuscuta

1. These are non-chlorophyll bearing leafless, twining parasitic seed plants, they attach to the host.
2. They are yellow, pink or orange in colour.
3. The initial appearance of parasite in field is noticed as small masses of branched, thread like, leafless stem, which are devoid of green pigment and twice around the stem or leaves of the hosts.
4. The leaves are represented by minutes functionless scales.
5. When the stem of parasites comes in contact with the hosts, the minute root like organs, haustoria penetrates into the host cortex and serves as an organ of food absorption.
6. When the relationship with the host is firmly established, the dodder plant losses the contact from soil.
7. The flowers are found in clusters, they are tiny, white, pink or yellowing in colour.
8. The seeds are formed in capsule. A single plant may produce as many as 3000 seeds.
9. The common dodder *Cuscuta granovil* attacks clovers, berseem flag and many other oilseed crops. It also attacks ornamental and hedge plants. It is fast developing parasites and within 2-3 seasons may destroy a complete plant.

10. The dodder perepetuates through seeds which remain dormant in the soil unitl favourable seasons returns, stem portion of parasite is also meant of perpetuation.

Management

1. Selection of dodder free seeds for sowing.
2. Crop rotation with non host plants.
3. Restriction of flow of irrigation water through infected field.
4. Dodder can be controlled by the use of soil herbicides, such as chloroproopham, dichobhil, donoseb, DCPA, glyphosate, these chemicals kills the dodder plant upon its germiantion from seed.
5. Preventing the movement of grazing animals from infected field to clean field.

Partial Root Parasite - Striga

Family: Scrophulariaceae

Genus: Striga (Witch weed)

1. Striga is well known partial root parasite of sugarcane, cereals, jawar, maize, and millets in India.
2. There are four species of Striga reports in the country on sugarcane, rice , sorghum and other millets like *S.lutee S.densiflora , S. quphrasioldes, S.asiatica.*
3. These plants although obligate parasites do not obtain all of their nutrient material from their host root. They posses' chlorophyll bearing leaves.
4. Striga can be found on light as well as heavy soil in rabi and kharif season. The seeds of Striga are very minute and produced in great abundance 50,000 to 1, 00,000 seeds /pl/yr.
5. One flower / capsule contains 1200-1500 seeds.
6. Viability of those seeds has been reported to be from 12-40 years. Short distance dissemination of these seeds.
7. For germination of seeds of Striga species, stimulant provided by the root executes of specific host is essential.
8. Seed starts germination after 7-10 days. After germination, the parasites grow below the soil surface for about 4-8 weeks and produces underground stem and root.
7. The underground portion of the stem contains bud in the axil of leaf.

8. Stem of parasite forms haustoria which penetrates the root of hosts plants and also water and nutrient eventually wasting and destroying the host.

Management of Striga

1. Deep ploughing after harvest reduces the vialibility of seed.
2. Complete eradication of parasite before flowering.
3. Regular Interculture should be followed.
4. Crop rotation with Cotton-Jowar- Groundnut.
5. Weedicides are used to control Striga before flowering.
    - 2-4-D @ 2.5 lit/500 lit of H_2O per ha.
    - Attrazine @ 2 kg / 500 lit of water per ha.
    - . 1% TCPA @ 45 kg/ha.

Partial Stem Parasite - Loranthus or Bandgul

1. Loranthus is common parasites of mango trees.
2. In Northern India, 60-90% of mango trees and large no of other trees are heavily or moderately infected by these parasites.
3. Loranthus (*Dendrophthae falcate)*, the most common species in India is the semi parasitic of the tree trunk and branches. Their leaves posses chlorophyll and synthesize carbohydrate constituent of their food requirement.
4. The parasite attacks, the aerial parts of the host trees, by developing haustoria and obtain its nourishment directly from the vascular system of the host plant. The continuous sucking of the food material by parasite resulting the host to die.
5. Since the parasite attacks the aerial part of host tree, situated far above the soil level and as such devoid of root system of its own.
6. The flowers of parasites are borne in clusters. They are long tabular in shape and usually greenish, red or white in colour according to species.
7. The fruit is fleshy and contains a solitary seed. It is sweet eaten by birds and animals.
8. The parasite is spread by dispersal of its seed, mostly through birds and to some extent by other animals.
9. The damage done by the parasite is most marked in production of new growth of the host. Leaves are reduced in size and show unhealthy green colour. The quantity and yield of fruit is considerably lowered.

Management

1. Injection of CuSo4 or 2-4-D into the infected branches has been found effectively in eradicating the parasite from mango.
2. Scrapping of parasite before seedling from the infected bunches.
3. Sowing of branches sufficient low to the tumours.

Model Question Papers

A. Objective Types

a. Multiple Choice Questions

1. Sugarcane ratoon stunting is caused by
   (a) Phytoplasmas (b) Viroids
   (c) *Cavibacter xyli sub sp xyli* (d) Virus
2. Phytoplasmas contain
   (a) RNA only (b) DNA only
   (c) RNA+ DNA (d) RNA or DNA
3.Spiroplasma are mostly
   (a) Xylem inhibiting (b) Phloem inhibiting
   (c) Both (a) and ((b) (d) Stomata inhibiting
4. Potato spindle tuber disease is caused by
   (a) Viroid (b) Phytoplasma
   (c) Spiroplasma (d) Virus
5. Bacteriophage is
   (a) Naked single stranded RNA particle(b) A Virus infecting bacteria
   (c) A virus infecting eukaryotic cell (d) Animal virus
6. Bacteriophage word was given by
   (a) Mayer. (b) D'Herelle
   (c) Hashimoto (d) Doi *etal*
7. Cuscuta is a
   (a) Complete stem parasite (b) Complete root parasite
   (c) Semi stem parasite (d). Semi root parasite
8. Phloem necrosis of coffee is caused by–
   (a) MLO (b) Virus
   (c) Protozoa (d) Algae

9. Spiroplasma is inhibited by an antibiotic –
   (a) Penicillin (b) Tetracycline.
   (c) Streptocyclin (d) Aureofungin
10. The disease caused by Spiroplasma
   (a) Corn stunt (b) White bud of maize
   (c) Cirtus stubborn (d) All
11. Fastidious vascular bacteria are also called –
   (a) RLO (b) MLO
   (c) Viroids (d) Prion
12. RLO is usually transmitted by
   (a) Leaf hopper (b) White fly
   (c) Aphid (d) Thrips
13. The disease caused by Phytoplasma
   (a) Corn stunt (b) White bud of maize
   (c) Cirtus stubborn (d) Little leaf of brinjal
14. Fried egg' like colonies on agar medium is characteristic feature of
   (a) Phytoplasma (b) Spiroplasma
   (c) Viroid (d) Prion
15. Red rust of coffee is caused by
   (a) Phytoplasma (b) Spiroplasma
   (c) Viroid (d) Algae

Q. No	Answer	Q. No	Answer
1	(c) *Cavibacter xyli sub sp xyli*	9	(b) Tetracycline
2	(c) RNA+ DNA	10	(d) All
3	(b) Phloem inhibiting	11	(a) RLO
4	(a) Viroid	12	(a) Leaf hopper
5	(b) A Virus infecting bacteria	13	(d) Little leaf of brinjal
6	(b) D'Herelle	14	(a) Phytoplasma
7	(a) Complete stem parasite	15	(d) Algae
8	(c) Protozoa	16	

b. True/False

1) Orobanchea is a complete rot parasite.
2) Cuscuta is a complete stem parasite.

3) Striga is partial root parasite of sugarcane, cereals, jawar, maize, and millets in India.
4) Neamtode is triploblastic, bilaterally symmetrical, unsegmented, pseudocoelomate invertebrate.
5) Nematode lacks specialized organs for respiration and circulation.
6) The life cycle of a plant parasitic nematode has six stages.
7) The Mollicutes are a class of bacteria distinguished by the absence of a cell wall.
8) The genus Spiroplasma are helical and move by twisting .
9) Most of the important parasitic genera belong to the order Tylenchida .
10) When an ectoparasite feed at a particular site for a brief period and the move to the next site. It is called migratory ectoparasite.
11) Loranthus is common parasites of mango trees.
12) Witch weed posses' chlorophyll bearing leaves.
13) Endoparasites considered to be the most destructive forms of plant parasitic nematodes.
14) Meloidogyne is a sedentary endoparasites nematode.
15) Tylenchulus semipenetrans is a sedentary semi-endoparasite nematode.
16) Tylenchorhynchus is a migaratory semi-endoparasite.
17) Heterodera, and globodera are considered to be the most advanced plant parasitic nematodes.
18) The best known genus in mollicutes is *Mycoplasma.*
19) Phloem necrosis of coffee is caused by Protozoa.
20) Red rust of tea is caused by an algae.

Q. No	Answer	Q. No	Answer
1.	True	11	True
2.	True	12	True
3.	True	13	True
4.	True	14	True
5.	False	15	True
6.	True	16	True
7.	True	17	True
8.	True	18	True
9.	True	19	True
10.	True	20	True

Descriptive Questions

a. Short answer

1. What features are used for identification of plant parasitic nematodes?
2. The nematodes placed in which two class and order.
3. Write any three modes of feeding in plant nematodes.
4. Differentiate between holo and hemiparasites of higher plants.
5. Write down the significant feateures of Phytoplasma.
6. Why is the designation RLO now abondaned?
7. Why are aphids unable to transmit mollicutes?
8. Why are Phytoplasma and Liberatobacter treated as Candidatus genera?
9. Why are Phytoplasmas considered as basically insect parasites?

b. Long Answer

1. Write notes on
   i. Classification of plant parasitic nematodes
   ii. Under and above ground symptoms produced by nematodes
   iii. Integrated nematode management
2. Classify plant parasitic nematodes on the basis of their parasitism.
3. White down the symptoms and nature of damage caused by Heterodera, Meloidogyne and Anguina
4. Distinguish between
   i. Mycoplasma and Spiro plasma
   ii. Orbanchae and Striga
   iii. Host range and host preference of parasitic angiosperm.
5. Explain in brief about other plant pathogens: Mollicutes; Flagellant protozoa; FVB; Green algae and parasitic higher plants.

11

Viruses, Virus Transmission & Viroids

Definition of Virus

Viruses are very small (submicroscopic) infectious particles (virions) composed of a protein coat and a nucleic acid core. They carry genetic information encoded in their nucleic acid, which typically specifies two or more proteins. Translation of the genome (to produce proteins) or transcription and replication (to produce more nucleic acid) takes place within the host cell and uses some of the host's biochemical "machinery". Viruses do not capture or store free energy and are not functionally active outside their host. They are therefore parasites (and usually pathogens) but are not usually regarded as genuine microorganisms.

Mathwas (1981) considers a virus as a set of one or more template molecules normally encased in a protective coat or coats of protein or lipoprotein, which is able to organize its own replication only within suitable host cells where its production is:

i) Dependent on hosts protein synthesizing machinery (ribosomes).
ii) Organised from pools of required material rather than binary fission and
iii) Located at sites which are not separated from the host cell contents by a lipoprotein bilayer membrane.

Characteristic of Virus

1. Viruses contain a single type of nucleic acid, either RNA or DNA, never both.
2. The nucleic acid carries the genome of the virus which differs from one virus to another.
3. The genome in the nucleic acid strand directs the synthesis of specific proteins for the protein coat which must be present in all viruses throughout their active phase except at the time of replication when, protein coat and nucleic acid are separated
4. Viruses rely on living host cells for most of the enzymes necessary for their replication.

5. Because viruses lack the synthesis of the Lipman system, they are unable to multiply.

Nature of Virus

Each plant virus consists of two components the **nucleic acid** and the **protein coat** or capsid. The mature particle of a plant virus is generally called **virion** and the whole infective particle is called as **Nucleocapsid.**

Nucleic Acid of Viruses

1. Nucleic acid portion of the virus particle is called as **Genome**.
2. Genomes are organized as single nucleic acid molecules that are linear or circular.
3. They may have as few as four genes or as many as several hundred.
4. They may be double-stranded DNA, single-stranded DNA, double-stranded RNA, or single-stranded RNA.
5. Genome is actual infective component.
6. Majority of plant viruses contain RNA.
7. Some viruses (Cauliflower mosaic virus, , maize streak virus, mung bean yellow mosaic virus) contain DNA.
8. Most plant viruses contain single strand of RNA.
9. In double stranded viruses (as RNA or ds DNA) the two strands are coiled around each other helically.

The Virus Protein

1. Protein coat that encloses the viral genome is called **capsid.**
2. Its structure may be rod-shaped, polyhedral, or complex.
3. Composed of many **capsomeres,** protein subunits made from only one or a few types of protein.
4. It helps viruses infect their host.
5. It protects nucleic acid (RNA or DNA) of virus.
6. It is made-up of different amino acid sequences in different viruses.
7. Protein shell or coat protects viral nucleic acid from environment.

Different types of viruses

The following are the examples for different types of viruses

Sl.No	Types		Examples
1. RNA viruses			
	a. Single stranded	With one segment	Tobacco mosaic viruses Lettuce necrotic yellow virus
		With two segments	Cowpea mosaic virus Tobacco ring spot virus
		With three segments	Cucumber mosaic virus
		With more number of segments	Potato virus x Tomato spotted wilt virus
	b. Double stranded		Wound tumour virus Fiji disease virus Reo virus
2. DNA viruses			
	Double stranded		Cauliflower mosaic virus
	Single stranded		Maize streak virus, ϕX174

3. Satellite Viruses

These arc viruses associated with certain typical viruses but depend on the latter for multiplication and plant infection and reduce the ability of the typical viruses act like parasite of the associated typical virus.

4. Helper viruses

The viruses which help multiplication of satellite RNA are called helper viruses.

5. Virusoids

These are viriod like, small, single stranded , circular RNAs that are present inside some RNA viruses, virusides are the part of genetic material of these viruses and therefore , form an obligatory association with these viruses so that neither the virus not the virosoid can multiply and infect a plant in the absence of its partner.

6. Temperate viruses

Viruses that can integrate their genome into a host chromosome and remain latent until they initiate a lytic cycle.

8. Provirus

Viral DNA that inserts into a host cell chromosome.

9. Retrovirus (Retro = backward):

RNA virus that uses reverse transcriptase to transcribe DNA from the viral RNA genome.

9. Viroid

These are small (250-400 nucleotide), naked, single stranded, circular RNAs capable of causing disease in plants by themselves.

Morphology of Viruses

Plant viruses are usually described as

1. Elongated (Rigid rod or Flexious thread)

S.No	Morphology	Example	Size(nm)
1	Rigid rod	Barley stripe mosaic virus	20X 10
		Tobacco mosaic virus	15 X 300
2	Flexuous thread	Potato virus X	10-13 X480
		Citrus tristeza virus	10-14 X 2000

2. Spherical (Isometric or Polyhedral) :

All spherical viruses are actually polyhedral ranging in diameter about 17 nm to 60 nm. Examples;

Sl.No	Example	Diameter (nm)
1	Tobacco necrosis satellite virus	17
2	Wound tumour virus	60
3	Tomato spotted wilt virus	70-80

3. Rhabdo Viruses

These are short bacillus like rods approximately 3 to 5 times as long as they are wide.

S.No	Example	Diameter (nm)
1	Potato yellow dwarf virus	75X 380 nm.
2	Wheat striate mosaic virus	65X 270 nm.
3	Lettuce necrotic yellow virus	52 X 300 nm.

Classification of Plant Viruses

Internatiponal committee on taxonomy of viruses has classified viruses into different groups. The classification is based on particle morphology and size, naked or enveloped ncleocapsids, number of virion types, number of genome fragements, type of nucleic acid and strandness of nucleic acid.The group name is is mostly based on the type virus included in the group.

Group	Name	Pieces of RNA/DNA	Shape
ssRNA			
Bromovirus	*Brome mosaic virus* *Dahlia mosaic virus*	ssRNA	Elongated
Carlavirus	*Carnation latent virus*	ss RNA	Elongated
Closterovirus	*Beet yellow virus*	ssRNA	Elongted
Comovirus	*Cow pea mosaic virus*	ssRNA	Isomtric
Cucumovirus	*Cucumber mosaic virus*	ssRNA	Isomtric
Dianthovirus	*Carnation ring spot virus*	ssRNA	Isomtric
Geminivirus	*Maize streak virus*	ssRNA	Isomtric
Hordei virus	*Barley stripe mosaic virus*	ssRNA	Elongated
Ilarvirus	*Tobacco streak virus*	ssRNA	Isomtric
Luteovirus	*Barley yellow dwarf virus*	ssRNA	Isomtric
Nepo virus	*Tobacco ring spot virus*	ssRNA	Isomtric
Potyvirus	*Pototo virus x*	ssRNA	Elongated
Rhabdovirus	*Lettuce necrotic mosaic virus*	ss RNA	Baciliformed
Sobemovirus	*Southern bean mosaic virus*	ssRNA	Isomtric
Tobamo virus	*Tobacco mosaic virus*	ssRNA	Elongated
Tobravirus	*Tobaco rattle virus*	ssRNA	Elongated
Tymovirus	*Turnip yellow mosaic virus*	ssRNA	Isomtric, Elongated
Tombus virus	*Tomato bushy stunt virus*	ssRNA	Isomtric,
dsRNA			
Fiji virus	*Fiji disease virus*	dsRNA	Isomtric
Phytoreovirus	*Wound tumor virus*	dsRNA	Isomtric
Orizavirus	*Rice ragged stunt virus*	dsRNA	Isomtric
Alphacryptovirus	*White clover cryptic virus 1*	dsRNA	Isomtric
Betacryptovirus	*White clover cryptic virus 1*	dsRNA	Isomtric
Varicosavirus	*Lettuce big vein associated virus*	dsRNA	Rod shaped
Endornavirus	*Vicia faba endornavirus*	dsRNA	Unknown
ss DNA			
Mastrevirus	*Maize streak virus*	ssDNA	Isomtric
Curtovirus	*Beet curly top virus*	ssDNA	Isomtric
Topocuvirus	*Tomato pseudo curly top virus*	ssDNA	Isomtric
Begomovirus	*Bean golden mosaic virus* *Mung bean yellow mosaic virus* *Tobacco and Tomato leaf curl virus* *Soybean leaf curl virus*	ssDNA	Isomtric

Group	Name	Pieces of RNA/DNA	Shape
Nanovirus	*Subterranean clover stunt virus*	ssDNA	Isomtric
Babuvirus	*Banana bunchy top virus*	ssDNA	Isomtric
ds DNA			
Caulimovirus	*Cauliflower mosaic virus* *Dahalia mosaic virus*	ds DNA	Isomtric
Soymovirus	*Soybean chlorotic mottle virus*	ds DNA	Isomtric
Cavemovirus	*Cassava vein mosaic virus*	ds DNA	Isomtric
Petu virus	*Petunia vein clearing virus*	ds DNA	Isomtric
Cheravirus	*Cherry rasp leaf virus*	ds DNA	Isomtric
Badnavirus	*Commelina yellow mottle virus*	ds DNA	Baciliformed
Tungrovirus	*Rice tungro bacilliform virus*	ds DNA	Baciliformed

Symptoms of Plant Viruses

Symptoms are the expression of the diseased condition of the plant. All most all virus disease seem to cause some degree of reduction in yield and the length of life of virus infected plants is usually shortened. The most obvious symptoms of virus infected plants are usually those appearing on the leaves but some viruses may cause striking symptoms on the stem, fruits and roots.

Symptoms

I) External (Macroscopic)

(a) Local

These are the symptoms produced at the site of artificial inoculation on leaves with virus.

i) **Chlorotic local lessions**: Infect cell loose chlorophylls and other pigments. For example, TMV on Cowpea host.

ii) **Necrotic local lessions**: Infect cell die. For example, TMV on *Nicotina glutinosa* host.

iii) **Ring spot local lesions**: Consist of central group of died cells near inoculated area (Necrotic ring) For example, Potato Virus: on *Chenopodium amaranticolar* host.

B) Systemic

The virus is found throughout the plant in practically all plant viruses that appear in the field.

(a) Colour Breaking (Variegation)

i) Mosaic

Mosaic are characterized by non uniform foliage coloration, with a more or less distinct intermingling of normal and light green or yellowish patches. Mosaic type symptoms may be described as follows.

a. Streak or stripe: Red stripe of jowar.
b. Vein clearing: BCMV.
c. Vein banding: Beat curly top.
d. Inter veinal mosaic light discolouration restricted in between veins.

ii) Mottling

If the discoloured patch of a variegated leaves are rounded the variegation is usually designated as mottling.

iii) Line Pattern

a. Oak leaf pattern (OLP) (Apple oak leaf)
b. Systemic Rings (AMV on tobacco)

b. Malformation

1. Change in leaf form, any deviation from normal.
2. This includes uneven growth of leaf lamina leaves becomes curled, britle (Crinkling) and show, prominaces and depressions (puckering) upward and downward curling, vein distortion, leaf enation, galls and tumours.

c. Others

a. Reddening of leaves cotton red leaf due to abnormal accumulation of anthoecynamin.
b. Blackening of veins Potato virus 'Y' in potato (Due to more synthesis of melanis).
c. Bronzening: Example. TSWV, in Tomato
d. Etching: Tobacco etch virus.

II) Internal (Microscopic)

These include inclusion bodies. Inclusions are microscopic bodies produced by some of the viruses. These are produced in cytoplasm or nucleic acid.

(a) Cytoplasm

1. **Amorphous** or amoeboid also called as X-bodies produced by spherical or oval viruses Example. CMV.

2. **Crystalline:** These type of inclusions are produced by rod shaped viruses. Example. Red clover vein mosaic, Cactus virus, and Petunia ring spot.

b) **Nucleus**

Example. Tobacco etch virus, rectangular plates. BCMV- Strain pisum Virus -2. Isometric crystals.

Proliferation (Toratonic symptoms)

1. Asymmetry of leaf lamina. Example, Grape fan leaf.
2. Blistering: Dark green area may be raised to give blistering effect. Margin of leaves twisted Example. BCMV.
3. Tumours: Clover wound tumour virus.
4. Swelling of stem: Cocoa swollen shoot virus.
5. Flattening of branches and distribution of stem: Apple flat limb.
6. Enations: These are the out growth in different shape and form either on veins or leaf lamina.
7. Vein enation: Citrus onation virus, Pea enation mosaic.
8. Leaf enation: Cotton leaf curl: Tobacco leaf curl.
9. Galls: Woody galls of citrus.
10. Pitting: (a) Stem pitting – Apple stem pitting, Citrus twisteza virus on kagzi lime. b) Fruit pitting: Pear stony pit- Apple groove virus on apple.
11. Stunt: Tomato bushy stunt.
12. Dwarfing: Barley yellow dwarf.
13. Leaf roll: Potato leaf roll.
14. Yellows: Beet Yellows.
15. Pox: Plum pox virus.

Latent Viruses and Masked Symptoms

1. Latent Viruses:

Many viruses may infect certain hosts without ever causing development of visible symptoms on them. Such viruses are usually called as "**Latent viruses**" and hosts are called as "**Symptomless carriers**".

2. Masked Symptoms:

Virus induced plant symptoms that are absent under certain environmental conditions, but appear when the host is exposed to certain conditions of light and temperature.

Transmission of Plant Viruses

The plant virus rarely, if ever, come out of plant spontaneously. For this reason, Plant viruses are not disseminated as such by wind or water. Viruses are transmitted from plant to plant in a number of ways such as vegetative, propagation, mechanically through sap and by seed, pollen, insect, mites, nematodes, dodder and fungi.

1. Mechanical Transmissions

Such transmissions may takes place between closely spaced plants after a strong wind by contact , when plants are wounded during cultural operations, virus infected sap adhering to the tools, worker hands or cloth accidently transmitted to the subsequently wounded plants.Example, Potato virus: (PV-X,TMV on Tobacco and Tomato)

2. Transmission by Vegetative Propagation

Plants are propagated vegetatively by budding or grafting or by cutting or by the use of tubers, corms, bulbs or rhizome. Any virus present in the mother plant from which these organs are taken will almost always be transmitted to the progeny. Transmission of viruses may also occur through natural root grafts of adjacent plant.

3. Transmission by Seed and pollen

Plant virus transmission from generation to generation occurs in about 20% of plant viruses. When viruses are transmitted by seeds, the seed is infected in the generative cells and the virus is maintained in the germ cells and sometimes, but less often, in the seed coat. When the growth and development of plants is delayed because of situations like unfavourable weather, there is an increase in the amount of virus infections in seeds. There does not seem to be a correlation between the location of the seed on the plant and its chances of being infected. Little is known about the mechanisms involved in the transmission of plant viruses via seeds, although it is known that it is environmentally influenced and that seed transmission occurs because of a direct invasion of the embryo via the ovule or by an indirect route with an attack on the embryo mediated by infected gametes. These processes can occur concurrently or separately depending on the host plant. It is unknown how the virus is able to directly invade and cross the embryo and boundary between the parental and progeny generations in the ovule. Many plants species can be infected through seeds including but not limited to the Leguminosae, Solanaceae, Compositae, Rosaceae, Cucurbitaceae, Gramineae. Bean common mosaic virus is transmitted through seeds.

4. Dodder Transmission

Dodder (Cuscuta spp.) is a parasitic plant that can transmit viruses from infected plants to healthy plants. Dodder does this by establishing a vascular connection with the host plant, allowing the virus to pass through the plant's vasculature.

How does fodder transmit viruses?

Dodder winds around the host plant. The dodder's haustoria penetrate the host plant's tissue. The haustoria establish cellular connections with the host plant. If the host plant is infected with a virus, the virus particles are taken up by the haustoria. The virus particles are transmitted to another host plant through the dodder.

Examples of viruses transmitted by dodder

I. Cucumber mosaic virus.
II. Tobacco mosaic virus
III. Potato stem mottle virus.
IV. Beet curly top virus.
V. Tomato bushy stunt virus.
VI. Tobacco rattle virus.

5. Natural Modes of Transmission

This includes air borne transmission through insects and mites and soil borne transmission through nematodes and fungus.

(a) Air Borne through Insects

The most common and important means of virus transmission in the field.

Members of the order Homoptera- Aphids, Jassids, Leaf hopper, white flies, mealy bug , scale insects.

Thysanoptera – Thrips, coleopteran- Beetles.

Insects with sucking mouth parts carry plant viruses on their stylet- stylet borne or non persistances.

b) Circulative

1. Circulative Viruses (Persistent)

A circulative virus is one that passes into a vector through the mouth parts, circulates internally and enlarges through the salivary glands.

2. Propagative Viruses

Propagative viruses are those viruses which multiply in their insect vectors and transmit them for a long time but very often for as long as they live.

C) Insect Vectors

Virus transmitting insect is called vector. Viruses are mostly really on insect for transmission (400 species of insect vector transmitting more than 200 viruses).The viruses are transmitted by diffeent types of insects and most efficient vectors are of sucking and bitting type of insects.

a. **White Flies:** Yellow vein of okra, Tobacco leaf curl, Pumpkin yellow mosaic , Mung yellow mosaic, Sweet potato mosaic,Cotton leaf curl, Cassava mosaic.
b. **Aphids:** These are the most important insect vector of plant viruses and transmit great majority (about 170) of the all stylet borne viruses Example. Soybean mosaic, Pea enation mosaic, Lettuce necrotic, Yellows borne mosaic, Potato leaf roll, Red clover mosaic, MCMV, AMV, BYMV.
c. **Leaf Hoppers:** All leaf hoppers transmitted viruses are circulatory, several are known to multiply in the vector (propagative), cause disturbance an phloem region Example, Rice tungro viruses, Rice, dwarf viruses, Potato yellow dwarf ,Maize mosaic, Beet curly top, Maize rough dwarf.
d. **Thrips:** Tomato spotted wilt virus.
e. **Beetles:** Cowpea mosaic virus, Bean pod mottle, Squash mosaic, Cowpea chlorotic motile virus, Raddish mosaic.
f. **Mites:** Transmit viruses like Pigeonpea sterility mosaic, Peach mosaic, Fig mosaic, Wheat streak mosaic.

D. Nematodes

Hewitt and colleagues (1958)first showed that Fan leaf virus of grapevines is transmitted by dagger nematode, *Xiphinema index*. Later, a few other plant viruses were reported to be transmitted by nematodes and now abou 24 plant viruses are known to be transmitted by neamtodes.Most nematodes parasitic on green plants belong to order Tymenchyda, but noen of this group has yet been found to be a vector virus. All species of nematodes known to transmit viruses are members of the order Dorylaimida and belong to the five genera: *Xiphineama, Longidorus, Paralongidorus, Trichodorus* and *Paratrichodorus.* Approximately 20 plant viruses have been shown to be transmitted by one or more species of 4 genera of soil inhabiting Ectoparasitic Nematodes. Examples of viruses that can be transmitted by nematodes are given below.

Sr.No	Group	Nematode Virus Vectors	Example
1	NEPO: Nematode transmitted polyhedral soil viruses	*Xiphinema index*	Grape vine fan leaf
		Xiphinema coxy	Cherry leaf roll
		Xiphinema americaum	Ring spot of tobacco, Tomato, Soybean bud blight, Bringal mosaic.
2	NETU: Nematode transmitted tubular soil viruses	*Longidours*	Rasberry ring spot, tomato black ring.
		Trichodours and Paratrichodorous	Rod shaped viruses, Tobacco rattle virus, Pea early browing virus

E. Fungus

Soil inhabiting speices of chytrid true fungi belonging to two genera *Olpidium* and *Synchitrium* and two species of protozoa (fungal like) belonging to two genera *Polymyxa* and *Spongospora* have been proved to be vectors of certain category of plant viruses. Examples of viruses that can be transmitted by fungi are given below.

Sr.No	Fungus Virus Vectors	Example
1	*Olpidium brassicae*	Lettuce big vein, Tobacco necrosis , Cucumeber, necrosis, Tobacco stunt virus
2	*Synchytrium endobioticum*	PU-X virus
3	*Polymyxa graminis*	Wheat mosaic virus, Beat necrotic yellow vein virus.
4	*Spongospora subteranea*	Potato mop top virus

Horizontal and Vertical Transmission of virus

Plant viruses spread from plant to plant by two major routes: horizontal transmission and vertical transmission.

Horizontal transmission = Route of viral transmission in which an organism receives the virus from an external source.

- Plants are more susceptible to viral infection if their protective epidermal layer is damaged.
- Insects may be *vectors* that transmit viruses from plant to plant and can inject the virus directly into the cytoplasm.
- By using contaminated tools, gardeners and farmers may transmit plant viruses.

Vertical transmission = Route of viral transmission in which an organism inherits a viral infection from its parent.

- Can occur in asexual propagation of infected plants (e.g., by taking cuttings)
- Can occur in sexual reproduction via infected seeds.

Relationship between insect vector and virus

The virus vector relationship varies widely depending upon the duration of the virus in the vector. In case of persistent viruses, the virus may simply circulate through the body of the vector or propagate also. Hence, this relationship can be classified as

Non-persistant transmission: Refers to vector trasmission of a virus where the vector quickly picks up virus particles on its mouthparts and is infective for a short period of time (hours).

Semi-pertsistant transmission: Refers to vector trasmission of a virus where virus particles enter the vectors foregut. In this case the vector also picks up the virus quicly but is infective for somewhat longer (days) than with non-persistant transmission.e.g., Beet yellow virus

Circulative transmission: Refers to vector trasmission of a virus where virus particles must circulate through the vectors hemolymph and enter the salivary glands to be tramsitted. In this case the vector aquisition and retention time is longer than with non or semi-persistant transmission.

Propagative transmission: Refers to vector trasmission of a virus where virus particles are repliacted in the the vector. In this case the vector retention time is longer than with circulative transmission and, in some cases, the virus can be transovarially transmitted.

Transovarial transmission: Refers to viral transmission from an insect vector to its offspring, meaning offpring of an infected vector are also infective.

Bacteriophages

Bacteriophage is a virus that infects bacteria.Very often the shortened form '*phage*' is used. Phages are ultramicroscopic agents that can pass through bacterial proof filter and infects bacteria.Phages are ubiquitous in nature and known to parasitise bacteria from all diverse habitates, such as soil, marine water, plants , intestines of animals.

Structure of T-even phage

A complete virion of T- even phage consists of the following structural units.

1. **Polyhedral head:** The head consists of an outer protein capsid enclosing genetic material or genome. The genome of a phage may contain ssRNA, dsRNA, ssDNA, or dsDNA.The phage genome is between 5 to 500 Kb long with either circular or linear arrangement.
2. **Collar:** The region between head and tail is reffered as collar.
3. **Helical tail:** The helical proteinaceous tail is attached with the head.The tail serves as organ of attachment or adsorption.

4. **Sheath:** In some phages the helical tail is covered by a sheath. The sheath provides a protective.
5. **Base plate:** It provides the support to the tail pins.
6. **Tail fibres:** There are tail fibres surrounding the tail. The tail fibres also helps in attachment process during host infection.
7. **Tail pins:** The tail pins are attached to the base plate connected to the tail and helps in attachment process.

Management of Plant Viruses

1. **Selection of Seed:** Select seed from disease free localities.
2. **Selection of Planting Materials:** Cutting, bull, rhizomes, tubers etc should be free from disease.
3. **Soil Fumigation:** Nematodes transmitted viruses can be reduced by the soil fumigation to control nematodes.
4. **Eradication:** Eradication of diseased plant to eliminate the inoculum from the field.
5. **Indexing:**Periodical indexing of the mother plants, producing propagative organs is necessary to ascertain these continuous freedom from virus.
6. **Protection against Insect Vectors:** This can be done by growing trap crops to check the insect vectors. Ex. Cotton reddening, White flies in bhendi.
7. **Weeds:** Removal and destruction of weeds that serve as host, broad leaf weeds in banana, orchard reduce bunchy tops.
9. **Use of Resistant Varieties:** Example. Parbhani Kranti is a vareity of bhendi that is resistant to yellow vein mosaic.
10. **Immunization:**The disease caused by severe strains of virus can be avoided if the plants are inoculated first with a mild strain of some viruses. e.g. Citrus greening.
11. **Temperature Treatment:** Sugarcane mosaic can be destroyed or reduce by hot water treatment 52 °C for 30 minutes.
12. **Use of Insecticides:** Control of insect vector with the use of insecticides like Thiomethoxam, Imidacloropid, Rogor etc.
13. **Quarantine Laws:** The best way to control virus disease is to keep it out of an area through a system of quarantine, inspections and certifications.

Viroids

Defnition

Viroid is circular, encapsulated, low molecular weight ($1.1\text{-}1.3x10^5$), self replicating, highly infectious ssRNA molecules.

General Characters

1. The viroid exists in *in vivo* as unencapsidated RNA.
2. They never contain any protein coat(capsid).
3. Genome of the viriod naked, single stranded RNA with 250-400 nucleotide, either linear or mostly circular. Viroids are smaller in size than viruses i.e 50 nm or 1.1 to 1.3 X 10^3 molecular weight.
4. Despited its small size, the infectious RNA is replicated autonomously in susceptible cells; that is, no helper virus is required for multiplication.
5. The infectious RNA consistas of one molecular species only.
6. Viroids are not able to synthesis protein and replicase enzyme required for replication.
7. Viroids replicate by direct RNA, copying in which all components required for viroid multiplication including RNA polymerase are provided by the host.
8. They cause diseases only in plants.
9. Viroids concentration and translocation is higher in growing parts of the plants (up to 0.2 mm from the apex).
10. Most of the types of symptoms observed with viral diseases also occurs viroids like epinasty, leaf distortions, vein clearing, localized chlorotic or necrotic spots, mottling of leaves, necrosis of leaves, and death of the whole plants.

Transmission

1. All known viroids are transmissible by mechanical means, either readily or with some difficulty.
2. Fram implements can result in mechanical transmission and spread of viroid infection is best possible by contact which consequently mainly responsible for the spread of the disease in nature.
3. Similarly, mechanical transmission and spread of viroid infection is best possible by using contaminated budding knives and other tools.
4. *Potato spindle tuber viroid*, *Chrysanthemum stunt viroid* and *Chrysanthemum chlorotic mottle viroid* are transmitted through sap

quite easily while others such as *Citrus exocortis* viroid is transmitted through sap with some difficulty.

5. Viroids those causing *Potato spindle tuber*, *Coconut cadang- cadang*, *Tomato bunchy top,* and apple scar skin disease appears to be transmitted through the pollen and seed.

Example

(i) Potato spindle tuber viroid.
(ii) Coconut cadang- cadang viroid.
(iii) Citrus exocortis viroid.
(iv) Chrysanthemum stunt viroid.
(v) Tomato bunchy top viroid.
(vi) Hot stunt viroid.
(vii) Avocardo sunblotch viroid.
(viii) Peach latent mosic viroid.

Management of viroid diseases

1. Use of viroid free propagating stocks.
2. Removal and destruction of viroid infected plants and following sanitary measures.
3. Washing of hands or sterilizing of tools after handling is very important aspect for viroid disease management.
4. Tools shoul be disinfected by dipping in a 10-20% sodium hypochlorite solution.
5. Mild strains of viroids are reported to proect the plants from effect of super infection with a severe strain of the same viroid.
6. No chemical are known to inhibit viroid infection.

Model Question Papers

A. Objective Types

a. Multiple Choice Questions

1. Bacteriophage contains

(a) ds DNA (b) ss DNA
(c) dsRNA (d) ss RNA

2. Which among the following virus contains single stranded DNA

(a) Gemini virus (b) Como virus
(c) Furo virus (d) Tobra virus

3. Mad cow disease is caused by
   (a) Virion (b) Prion
   (c) Bacteria (d) MLO
4. Virus contains single stranded DNA
   (a) Maize streak virus (b) Wound tumour virus
   (c) Tobacco ring spot virus (d) Cucumber mosaic virus
5. Sterility mosaic disease of pigeonpea spread by
   (a) Virus (b) Aphid
   (c) Whitefly (d) Mites
6. Virus contains double stranded RNA
   (a) Lettuce necrosis virus (b) Wound tumour virus
   (c) Tobacco ring spot virus (d) Cucumber mosaic virus
7. Which phage is called Lysogenic cycle
   (a) Virulent phage (b) Temperate phage
   (c) Lytic phage (d) Aseptic phage
8. The viruses which are usually helped or accompanied by smaller spherical particles of another serologically unrelated virus known as–
   (a) Satellite virus (b) Gemini viruses
   (c) Viroid (d) Capsid
9. Which among the following characteristics shows that viruses are non living entity
   (a) Multiply enormously (b) Obligate parasite
   (c) Mutate (d) Crystallized
10. Mostly Viruses contain–
   (a) RNA (b) DNA
   (c) Both RNA and DNA (d) Either RNA or DNA
11. NEPO virus is transmitted by
   (a) *Xiphinema index* (b) *Olpidium brassicae*
   (c) *Synchytrium endobioticum* (d) *Longidourus*
12. NEPTU virus is transmitted by
   (a) *Xiphinema index* (b) *Olpidium brassicae*
   (c) *Synchytrium endobioticum* (d) *Longidourus*
13. Potato mop top virus is transmitted by
   (a) *Xiphinema index* (b) *Olpidium brassicae*
   (c) *Synchytrium endobioticum* (d) *Spongospora subteranea*

14. Rice tungro viruses is transmitted by
    - (a) White flies
    - (b) Aphids
    - (c) Leaf hoppers
    - (d) Thrips

15. Refers to viral transmission from an insect vector to its offspring,
    - (a) Semi-pertsistant transmission
    - (b) Circulative transmission
    - (c) Propagative transmission
    - (d) Transovarial transmission

Answer

Q. No	Answer	Q. No	Answer
1	(a) ds DNA	9	(d) Crystallized
2	(a) Gemini virus	10	(a) RNA
3	(b) Prion	11	(a) *Xiphinema index*
4	(a) Maize streak virus	12	(d) Longidourus
5	(d) Mites	13	(c) *Spongospora subteranea*
6	(b) Wound tumour virus	14	(d) Leaf hoppers
7	(b) Temperate phage	15	(d) Transovarial transmission
8	(a) Satellite virus		

b.True /False

1. Viral replication is the formation of biological viruses during the infection process in the target host cells.
2. Viruses multiply only in living cells.
3. Majority of plant viruses contain RNA .
4. Hewitt and colleagues first showed that Fan leaf virus of grapevines is transmitted by dagger nematode, *Xiphinema index*
5. Mung bean yellow mosaic virus contain RNA.
6. Lipman system is absent in viruses.
7. Most DNA viruses assemble in the nucleus while most RNA viruses develop solely in cytoplasm.
8. Wound tumour virus contains double stranded RNA.
9. A circulative virus is one that passes into a vector through the mouth parts, circulates internally and enlarges through the salivary glands.
10. Mungbean yellow mosaic virus is transmitted by white fly.
11. Aphids are the most important insect vector of plant viruses.
12. Soybean mosaic virus is transmitted by aphid.
13. Pigeonpea sterility mosaic virus is transmitted by mite.
14. Lettuce big vein virus is transmitted by *Olpidium brassicae*.

15. The viruses which help multiplication of satellite RNA are called helper viruses.

Q. No	Answer	Q. No	Answer
1	True	9	True
2	True	10	True
3	True	11	True
4	True	12	True
5	False	13	True
6	True	14	True
7	True	15	True
8	True		

B. Desctiptive Questions

a. Short answer

1. Define Virus, Viroid & Prions.
2. Horzontal and vertical transmission of virus.
3. Differenciate between non-persistant transmission and semi-pertsistant Transmission.
4. Mechanism of plant virus transmission by vectors.
5. Ultra structural changes in plant due to virus infection.

b. Long answer

1. Short notes
   a. Replication of plant virus.
   b. Variability in plant virus.
2. Write notes on any of the four i.Geminiviruses II. Majro group of viruses III. Segmented viral genomes IV. dsDNA plant viruses.
3. Differentiate between i. Viruses and Viroids ii.Satellite virus and Satellite nucleic acids iii.Viroids and Prions.
4. Describe transmission of plant viruses?
5. Explain Virus vector relationship.
6. Classify plant viruses on the basis of nucleic acid with suitable examples.
7. Write an essay on management of plant viruses.
8. Describe the transmission of plant viruses by any four of the following
   i. Aphids ii White flies iii.Thrips iv. Beetles v. Planthoppers.

12

Principles of Plant Disease Control

Introduction

The goal of plant disease management is to reduce the economic and aesthetic damage caused by plant diseases. Conventionally, this has been called plant disease control, but current social and environmental values believe "control" as being absolute and the term too rigid. More multifaceted approaches to disease management, and integrated disease management, have resulted from this shift in attitude, however. Single often severe measures such as pesticide applications, soil fumigation or burning are no longer in common use. Further, disease management measures are often determined by disease forecasting or disease modeling rather than on either a calendar or prescription basis. Disease management might be viewed as proactive whereas disease control is reactive, although it is often difficult to distinguish between the two concepts, especially in the application of specific measures.

Plant disease management practices rely on anticipating occurrence of disease and attacking vulnerable points in the disease cycle (i.e., weak links in the infection chain). Therefore, correct diagnosis of a disease is necessary to identify the pathogen, which is the real target of any disease management program. A thorough understanding of the disease cycle, including climatic and other environmental factors that influence the cycle, and cultural requirements of the host plant, are essential to effective management of any disease.

The many strategies, tactics and techniques used in disease management can be grouped under one or more very broad principles of action. Differences between these principles often are not clear. The simplest system consists of two principles, prevention (prophylaxis in some early writings) and therapy (treatment or cure).The first principle (prevention) includes disease management tactics applied **before** infection (i.e., the plant is protected from disease), the second principle (therapy or curative action) functions with any measure applied **after** the plant is infected (i.e., the plant is treated for the disease). An example of the first principle is enforcement of quarantines to prevent introduction of a disease agent (pathogen) into a region where it does not occur. The second principle is illustrated by heat or chemical treatment of vegetative material such as bulbs, corms, and woody cuttings to eliminate fungi, bacteria, nematodes or viruses that are established within the plant material. Chemotherapy is the application of chemicals to an infected or diseased plant that stops (i.e., eradicates) the infection. There are five general disease control principles, avoidance exclusion, eradication, protection and resistance since plants do not have an immune system in the same sense as animals). These principles have been expanded or altered to some extent by others. They are still valid and are detailed

Principles of Plant Disease Management

Principles of plant disease management include

1. **Prophylaxis** (preventive)
   - Avoidance
   - Exclusion
   - Eradication
   - Protection
2. **Immunization**
   - Genetic resistance
   - Therapy (Physical therapy and chemical therapy)

1. **Avoidance of pathogen** :Avoiding disease by planting at times when or where inoculum is absent or ineffective due to unfavorable environment conditions.
   - Choice of geographic area
   - Selection of field
   - Choice of time of sowing
   - Disease escaping varieties
   - Selection of seed and planting stock
   - Modification of cultural practices

1. **Exclusion of inoculum** :Preventing the inoculum from entering or establishing in the field or area where it does not exist.
   - Seed treatment
   - Inspection and certification
   - Quarantine
   - Eradication of insect vectors

3. **Eradication of pathogens** :Reducing, inactivating, eliminating or destroying inoculum at the source, either from a region or from an individual plant in which it is already established.

- Biological control of plant pathogen
- Crop rotation
- Removal or destruction of diseased plant organs
- Rouging
- Eradication of alternate and collateral hosts
- Sanitation
- Heat and chemical treatment of disease plants
- Soil treatments

4. **Immunization**: It involves the modification of certain physical or physiological character(s) of the host such that it can repel infection or can reduce disease development or can minimize damage caused by the pathogen. The methods used are
   - Use of resistant varieties
   - Cross-protection

Cross protection refers to the protection of a plant by use of a mild strain of a pathogen against a virulent strain of the same pathogen that can cause more severe symptoms and damage. The method is generally used for viral disease management.

Disease resistance: Altering the effectiveness of the pathogen by selection or introduction of resistance genes in the plant.

- Selection and hybridization for disease resistance
- Resistance through chemotherapy
- Resistance through host nutrition

5. **Protection measures**: Preventing infection by creating a chemical toxic barrier between the plant and the pathogen is comes under protection measures

- Chemical treatment
- Chemical control of insect vectors
- Modification of environments

6. **Therapy**: Reducing severity of disease in an infected individual

- Chemotherapy
- Heat therapy
- Tree surgery

Strategy of disease management

It is well accepted that complete eradication of a pathogen from the earth of the ecosystem is very difficult. They are also intimate part of the ecosystem as human beings, animals and plants. Therefore; complete eradication is against the law of nature. The strategy for management lies on a amending the methods of cultivation through supplementary treatments, which can compensate for the upsetting of the natural ecosystem. The strategy should be to reduce the population of pathogen below permissible level so they do not cause damage. Keeping this in mind, the strategy of disease management should integrate all known methods taking into account the following factors.

1. Pathogen inhibition

As complete eradication of a pathogen is not possible, there should be more emphasis on management of its population. The pathogens will exist but control systems will have to be developed to maintain their population below the damaging level.

2. Tolerable losses

A few diseased seeds or plants are permissible in the field. If the loss is less, uprooting the diseased plants is more economical. In crops raised for seed two per cent disease infection is permissible, whereas in crops raised for consumption the permissible limit is 5 per cent.

3. Economical control

The strategy for disease management should be implemented after considering the cost benefit ratio. The return per unit of money spent must be sufficiently high.

4. Long term control

The strategy of disease management should attempt to utilize methods which have a long term effect so as to reduce the expenses and pollution of the environment.

5. Collective approach

Disease control cannot be achieved by a single farmer since pathogen can move from field to field. Hence, collective area wise approach is necessary for effective control.

One should always keep in mind that chemical control is a part of the strategy for disease management. Care should be taken not to accelerate the frequency of pesticide application. The use of chemical should be the last resort for controlling the diseases.

It is well known that any war cannot be won only on quantity of weapons available. Success only comes from a well planned strategy involving the best use of weapons in a coordinated manner at the right time and with proper methods. Similarly, the war against diseases can be won provided an integrated approach is employed and all the five basic factors discussed above are taken into account.

Model Practice Questions

A. Objective Questions

a. Multiple choice Questions

1. Avoiding disease by planting at times when or where inoculum is absent or ineffective due to unfavorable environment conditions.

   (a) Avoidance of pathogens (b) Exclusion of inoculum

   (c) Eradication of pathogens (d) Immunization

2. Preventing the inoculum from entering or establishing in the field or area where it does not exist.

   (a) Avoidance of pathogens (b) Exclusion of inoculum

   (c) Eradication of pathogens (d) Immunization

3. Reducing, inactivating, eliminating or destroying inoculum at the source, either from a region or from an individual plant in which it is already established.

   (a) Avoidance of pathogens (b) Exclusion of inoculum

   (c) Eradication of pathogens (d) Immunization

4. Preventing infection by creating a chemical toxic barrier between the plant and the pathogen is comes under protection measures

   (a) Avoidance of pathogens (b) Exclusion of inoculums

   (c) Eradication of pathogens (d) Protection

5. Disease management tactics applied before infection

   (a) Prevention (b) Cure

   (c) Regulation (d) Eradication

6. Disease management tactics applied after infection

   (a) Prevention (b) Cure

   (c) Regulation (d) Eradication

7. Avoidance of pathogen includes

(a) Choice of geographic area (b) Selection of field

(c) Disease escaping varieties (d) All

8. Exclusion of inoculum includes

(a) Seed treatment (b) Inspection and certification

(c) Quarantine (d) All

9. Reducing severity of disease in an infected individual

(a) Chemotherapy (b) Heat therapy

(c) Tree surgery (d) All

10. Altering the effectiveness of the pathogen by selection or introduction of resistance genes in the plant.

(a) Avoidance of pathogen (b) Exclusion of inoculums

(c) Eradication of pathogens (d) Disease resistance

Q. No	Answer	Q. No	Answer
1	Avoidance of pathogens	6	Cure
2	Exclusion of inoculum	7	All
3	Eradication of pathogens	8	All
4	Protection	9	All
5	Prevention	10	Disease resistance

b. True /False

1. Eradication of pathogens includes biological management of plant pathogens.
2. Plants with viral infections are rouged under the heading "Eradication of Pathogens."
3. Disease-escape variants fall under the category of pathogen avoidance.
4. Treatment with seeds is classified as inoculum exclusion.
5. The section on pathogen eradication includes quarantine.
6. The approach of cross protection is typically employed to manage viral diseases.
7. Disease management might be viewed as reactive approach.
8. Correct diagnosis of a disease is not necessary to identify the pathogen, which is the real target of any disease management program.
9. Chemotherapy is the application of chemicals to an infected or diseased plant that stops the infection.

10. Complete eradication of disease is against the law of nature

Q. No	Answer	Q. No	Answer
1	True	6	True
2	True	7	False
3	True	8	False
4	True	9	True
5	True	10	True

B. Descriptive Questions

a. Short answer

1. Write down the difference between control and management.
2. Prevention is better than cure prove with examples.
3. Why collective approach is very effective in management of plant diseases.
4. Explain immunization.
5. Explain disease escape.

b. Long answer

1. Distinguish between i.control and management ii. prevention and cure iii. Strategies vs tactics.
2. Why the term management is preferred over the term control?
3. Enlist principles of plant disease management.
4. Write down the major critical shortcoming of principles of plant disease management.
5. What is therapy.Name some fruit trees which can be controlled by tree therapy.
6. Discuss in details the general principles of plant disease management with suitable examples.
7. Elaborate strategies of plant disease management .
8. What is plant disease management? Give the basis of the principles of plant disease management.
9. Distinguish between the following: i. Exclusion and Eradication ii. Protectant and Eradicant iii. Prophylaxis and Immunization iv. Chemotherapy and Thermothearapy.

13

Physical Management

Principles

The principles involved in thermotherapy is that the pathogens present in seed material are inactivated or eliminated at temperatures nonlethal for the host tissues.The exact mechanism by which heat inactivates the pathogen is not fully understood. However, it is universally accepted that heat causes inactivation and not immobilization of the pathogen by heat. Th rate at which the pathogen is inactivated is determined by temperature, the higher the temperature, the faster is the inactivation. At constant temperature, the drop in the density of pathogenic inoculum.

Methods

Following physical methods are employed for reduction or elimination of primary inoculums that may be present in seed, soil, or planting material.

i. Hot water treatment (HWT)

Hot water treatment is widely used for the control of seed borne pathogens, especially bacteria and viruses. A list of various important diseases claimed to have been controlled by hot water treatment is given in Table-1.

Table-18.Control of seed borne pathogens through Hot –water treatment

Crop	Disease	Causal organism	Seed Treatment
Rice	White tip	*Aphlenchoides besseyi*	51-53°C for 15 min after dipping for 1 d in cool water.
	Udbatta	*Ehelis oryzae*	54°C for 10 min
Pearl millet	Downy mildew	*Sclerospora graminicola*	55°C for 10 min
Safflower	Leaf spots	*Alternaria spp.*	50°C for 30 min
Tomato	Black speck	*Pseudomonas syringae pv. tomato*	52°C for 1h
Cauliflower & Cabbage	Black rot	*Xanthomonas campestris pv. campestris*	50°C for 20 min
Tobacco	Hollow stalk	*Erwinia carotovora pv. carotovora*	50°C for 12 min.

Crop	Disease	Causal organism	Seed Treatment
Cluster bean	Blight	*Xanthomonas campestris pv. cyamopsidis*	56°C for 10 min
Sugarcane			**Setts Treatment**
	Red rot	*Colletotrichum falcatum*	54°C for 8 h
	Smut	*Ustilago scitaminea*	55 to 60°C
	Wilt	*Fusarium moniliforme*	50°C for 2 h
	Grassy shoot	MLO	54°C for 2h

The main drawback in the hot water treatment is that the seeds may be killed or loose its germ inability, if the period of treatment exceeds the specified time. So this method is replaced by other physical methods like Hot air and Aerated steam treatment wherein the seeds are exposed only to hot air/aerated steam.

ii. Hot air treatment (HAT)

Hot air treatment is less effective than hot water treatment but less injurious to seed and easy to operate. It has been used against several diseases of sugarcane. It is employed for treating canes which are soft and succulent. Hot air treatment at 54°C for 8h, effectively eliminates RSD pathogen without impairing the germination of buds. Similarly, grassy shoot disease of sugarcane has also been controlled by hot air at 54°C for 8 h.

iii. Steam and Aerated steam therapy (AST)

The use of aerated steam is more effective than hot air and safer than hot water in controlling seed borne infections. The heat capacity of water vapour is about half that of water and 2.5 that of air, hence air temperature and time required may be higher than that of hot water and lower than that of hot air. The advantages of this method include easier drying of seeds, low loss in germination, easy temperature control and no damage to seed coat of legumes. Sugarcane setts are also exposed to aerated steam at 50 °C for 3 hrs to eliminate mosaic virus.

iv. Moist hot air treatment (MHAT)

This method is effectively used in sugarcane to eliminate grassy shoot disease. Initially the setts are exposed to hot air at 54°C for 8 hrs, then exposed to aerated steam at 50 °C for 1 hr and finally to moist hot air at 54°C for 2 hours.

v. Solar heat treatment (SHT)

Solar heat treatment is effective in controlling both seed borne and soil borne diseases

a. Seed Borne Diseases

Solar heat treatment has been devised in India to eliminate the pathogen of loose smut of wheat. Luthra in 1953 devised a method to eliminate the deep seated infection of *ustilago nuda.* The method is popularly known as solar heat or solar energy treatment. In this method the seeds are soaked in cold water for 4 hours in the forenoon on a bright summer day followed by spreading and drying the seeds in hot sun for four hours in the afternoon. Then, the seeds are again treated with carboxin or carbendazin at 2g/kg and stored. This method is highly useful for treating large quantities of the seed lots.

b. Soil borne diseases

Soil Solarization

- Defined as hydrothermal treatment of soil for management of soil borne diseases.
- In this management tactics, the solar energy is preserved with the help of transparent polythene sheet for about 40 days to increase soil temperature (10-15^{0}C) above normal temperature enough to kill the most of the soil borne diseases.

Results of solarization

- Increased soil temperature.
- Improved soil physical and chemical features.
- Control of pests.
- Encouragement of beneficial soil organisms.
- Increased plant growth.
- Fungal diseases such as damping off, root and stem rots, wilt and blights diseases and some nematodes have been successfully managed by soil solarization.

Advantages

- Nonpesticidal and simple.
- No health or safety problems associated with use.
- No registration is required.
- Crops produced are pesticide-free and may command a higher.
- market price.
- Controls multiple soilborne diseases and pests.
- Selects for beneficial microorganisms.

- Tends to increase soil fertility.
- Increases soluble NO3, NH, Ca, Mg, K and soluble organic matter.
- May improve soil filth.
- Can speed up in-field composting of green manure.

Disadvantages

- It is restricted to areas with warm to hot summers.
- May be less effective in cooler coastal areas.
- Land must be taken out of production for 4 to 6 weeks during the summer.
- May not fit in with some cropping cycles.
- May be difficult for those using a small amount of land intensively.
- Limited number of retail outlets for UV-inhibiting plastics.
- Disposal may be a problem.
- Large amounts of plastic cannot currently be recycled in California.
- Some pests are not controlled or are difficult to control.
- No pest control in the furrows between strips (if applied in strip coverage).
- High winds and animals may tear the plastic.

vii. Refrigeration

The low temperature at or slightly above the freezing point checks the growth and activities of all such pathogens that cause a variety of post harvest diseases of vegetables and fruits. Therefore most perishable fruits and vegetables should be transported and stored in refrigerated vehicles and stores. Cool chains refrigerated space from field to consumer table is becoming very popular. Regular refrigeration is sometimes preceded by a quick hydro cooling or air cooling to remove the excess heat carried in them from the field to prevent development of new or latent infections.

viii. Radiation

Electromagnetic radiations such as ultraviolet (UV) light, x rays and y rays as well as particulate radiations have been studied in relation to management of post harvest diseases of horticultural crops. Gamma rays controlled post harvest fungal infections in peaches, straw berries and tomatoes but doses of radiation required to kill pathogens, were found injurious to host tissues. Some plant pathogenic fungi sporulate only when they receive light in the ultraviolet range. It has been possible to control diseases on green house vegetables caused by species of these fungi by covering or constructing the green house with a special UV absorbing vinyl film that blocks transmission of light wavelengths below 390 nm.

Model Practice Questions

A. Objective Questions

a. Multiple choice Questions

1. Management of plant diseases using physical means is called

(a) Cultural management (b) Physical management
(c) Biological management (d) Chemical management

2. The disease controls affected by physical practices are mostly

(a) Preventive (b) Curative
(c) Systemic (d) All

3. The principles involved in physical control or thermotherapy is that the pathogens present in seed, soil, or planting material.

(a) Are inactivated or eliminated at temperatures nonlethal for the host tissues.
(b) Heat causes inactivation and not immobilization of the pathogen by heat.
(c) The rate at which the pathogen is inactivated is determined by temperature, the higher the temperature, the faster is the inactivation.
(d) All

4 .Physical methods are employed for reduction or elimination of primary inoculums that may be present in

(a) Seed (b) Soil
(c) Planting material (d) All

5. Hot air treatment at which temperature effectively eliminates RSD pathogen without impairing the germination of buds.

(a) 54^0C for 8h (b) 50^0C for 8h
(c) 45^0C for 8h (d) 60^0C for 8h

6. Grassy shoot disease of sugarcane has also been controlled by hot air at .

(a) 54^0C for 8h (b) 50^0C for 8h
(c) 45^0C for 8h (d) 60^0C for 8h

7. Downy mildew disease of pearl millet has also been controlled by seed treatment with hot water at.

   (a) 55^0C for 10m (b) 50^0C for 10 min

   (c) 45^0C for 10 min (d) 60^0C for 10 min

8. Black rot disease of cabbage has also been controlled by seed treatment with hot air at .

   (a) 54^0C for 20min. (b) 50^0C for 20 min.

   (c) 45^0C for 20min. (d) 60^0C for 20min

9. Sugarcane setts are also exposed to aerated steam at what temperature to eliminate mosaic virus.

   (a) 54^0C for 3h (b) 50^0C for 3h

   (c) 45^0C for 3h (d) 60^0C for 3h

10. Solar heat treatment devised in India to eliminate the pathogen of which disease of wheat

    (a) Black rust (b) Brown rust

    (c) Yellow rust (d) Loose smut

11. Who devised a method in India to eliminate the deep seated infection of *ustilago nuda*

    (a) Blakeslee in 1953 (b) Luthra in 1953

    (c) Butler in 1955 (d) Vander plank 1955

12. Soil solarization results in

    (a) Increased soil temperature (b) Improved soil physical and chemical features

    (c) Control of pests (d) All

Q. No	Answer	Q. No	Answer
1	(b) Physical management	7	(a) 55^0C for 10m
2	(b) Curative	8	(b) 50^0C for 20 min
3	(d) All	9	(b) 50^0C for 3h
4	(d) All	10	(d) Loose smut
5	(a) 54^0C for 8h	11	(b) Luthra in 1953
6	(a) 54^0C for 8h	12	(d) All

b. True/False

1. Hot water treatment is widely used for the control of seed borne pathogens, especially bacteria and viruses.
2. The primary disadvantage of hot water treatment is that if the treatment period is prolonged beyond the allotted time, the seeds may be destroyed or lose their ability to germinate.

3. Hot air treatment is less effective than hot water treatment but less injurious to seed and easy to operate.
4. Hot air treatment has been used against several diseases of sugarcane and is employed for treating canes which are soft and succulent.
5. The use of aerated steam is less effective than hot air and safer than hot water in controlling seed borne infections.
6. Solar heat treatment is effective in controlling both seed borne and soil borne diseases.
7. Soil solarization is defined as hydrothermal treatment of soil for management of soil borne diseases.
8. Fungal diseases such as damping off, root and stem rots, wilt and blights diseases and some nematodes have been successfully managed by soil solarization
9. Hot air treatment is more effective than hot water treatment for disease managment but less injurious to seed and easy to operate.
10. Physical control is also called physical therapy or thermotherapy

Answer

Q. No	Answer	Q. No	Answer
1	True	6	True
2	True	7	True
3	True	8	True
4	True	9	False
5	False	10	True

2. Descriptive Questions

a. Objective questions

1. What is soil solarization?
2. What are the benefits of using solar energy for seed treatment?
3. How does hot water seed treatment work to eliminate pathogens?
4. When is the best time to perform soil solarization?
5. Why hot air treatment is less effective than hot water treatment.

b. Descriptive questions

1. What are the objectives of the physical methods of plant disease management? How are they helpful in minimizing plant disease?
2. Who developed solar heat treatment control? Name the disease for which the method was developed.

3. Write short notes on i.Principle of physical plant disease control ii.Hot water treatment iii. Hot air treatment iv.Steam and Aerated steam therapy
4. Explain about moist hot air treatment and solar heat treatment
5. Why aerated steam is more effective than hot air and safer than hot water in controlling seed borne infections?
6. What is soil solarization? Describe the method, advantage and disadvantage of soil solarization.
7. Describe the role of regrigeration and radiation in plant disease management.
8. What is physical control?. Write down the different physical methods used for plant disease control.
9. How can solar energy be used for the treatment of seeds? In which disease has it been used? Is it more coenveinet than chemical treatment.
10. Distinguish between hot water treatment and moist heat air treatment. Give atleast four examples of plant disease controlled by hot water treatment.
11. What is thermotheary ? What is the scientific principle involved in thermotherapy.

14

Cultural Management

Introduction.

The Cultural practices which includes manipulation /or adjustment of crop production techniques have been as old as possibly agriculture itself. In early stages of agriculture development, the growers through their experiences and observations had known that repeated cultivation of a particular crop species or variety on a piece of land often resulted in crop diseases. By proper crop rotations they had been avoiding such diseases. As a matter of fact, in the present day agriculture, cultural practices are being considered as essential backup methods for plant disease management. Cultural practices often offer the opportunity to alter the environment, the condition of the host, and/or the behavior of the causal agent, to achieve economic management of disease. Most cultural practices used to control plant disease are preventive in nature. Integration of cultural practices, host resistance and pesticides or biocontrol agents may be necessary to provide options for controlling economically important plant diseases.

Concept and Applications

Katan (1996) has divided cultural practices into three categories:

- Practices which are usually applied for agricultural purposes not related to crop protection, such as fertilization and irrigation. They may or may not have a positive or a negative side-effect on disease incidence.
- Practices which are used solely or mainly for disease control, such as sanitation for the eradication of infected plant residues, and flooding.
- Practices which are used for both agricultural purposes and disease control, such as crop rotation, grafting, and composting.

  The interest in studying the effect of cultural practices on disease has dual purpose: to develop suitable practices to control methods and to obtain information regarding their impact on diseases when they are used in agricultural practices in order to avoid negative side effects. Cultural practices must be employed, before or after planting. Deep ploughing and flooding are used before planting while irrigation and fertilization can be applied several times during the crop season for disease management.

Basic principles of cultural practices for disease control

The basic principles of cultural practices for disease control are

- Any potential control method may be considered, providing that it is environmentally, technologically and economically feasible
- Pesticide usage is minimized by combining with other non-chemical or chemical methods
- Diseases that are difficult to control or that involve problematic pesticides, e.g. methyl bromide, should be prioritized
- Economic aspects are taken into consideration.

The procedures for disease management through cultural practices

The procedures for disease management through cultural practices are described under the following three heads:

a. Production and use of pathogen free planting material.
b. Adjustment of cultural practices to minimize disease.
c. Sanitation.

A. Production and use of pathogen free planting material.

Many plant pathogens like bacteria, virus, fungi and nematodes are transmitted by diseased seed or other vegetative propagating parts. For successful disease control this source of primary inoculums must be destroyed. The following methods are followed to produce and use pathogen free seed material.

1. Proper drying and storage of seeds

If the seeds are not dried properly before storage they loose their germination capacity and also harbor several types of plant pathogen in it. The fungus, causing downy mildew of maize is found to be present in the seed when it is fresh. But when the seed is thoroughly dried the fungus present in it dies. Prolonged storage of seed also helps in eliminating several pathogens. *Fusarium solani f. sp. cucurbitae*, infecting cucurbits, is eliminated if the seeds are stored for two years before sowing. Similar eradication of pathogen has been achieved in anthracnose of cotton. Proper conditions of storage must be maintained avoid any harm to the seed.

2. Cleaning of seed

In many cases the pathogen is present in plant parts mixed with the seed. When such seed are used pathogen easily gets into the field. Thus, proper cleaning of seeds before sowing is essential. Common examples of diseases disseminated in this manner are ergot and smut of pearl millet, ear cockle of wheat, white rust of crucifers, ascochyta blight of chickpea, etc.

3. Adjustment of harvesting time

Disease incidence can be minimized by reducing spread of inoculums through adjustment of harvesting time and practice. For example, potatoes harvested when the tops are still green may easily get contaminated by late blight fungus present on the leaves. One of the practices to avoid tuber contamination or infection is to first remove the green tops and let them dry in the soil for 15 days before digging the tubers. When digging of tubers is prolonged the late blight fungus are killed and the produce becomes disease free.

4. Seed production areas

Seed should be produced in areas where the pathogens of major concerns are unable to establish or maintain themselves at critical levels during periods of seed development. Area with low relative humidity and low rainfall are favorable for production of high quality seeds. Some examples are bacterial blight of legumes, ascochyta blight of chickpea and anthracnose of cucurbits, etc. Such crops can be grown in dry areas with the help of irrigation.

5. Inspection of seed production areas

Periodical inspection of crops raised for seed production is an important procedure in the production of clean and healthy seeds. Destruction of diseased plants/organs at the time of inspection helps in reducing inoculums in the field and thus, the percentage of healthy seeds in the produce is increased. If disease incidence is high , the entire crop may be rejected for seed.

B. Adjustment of cultural practices to minimize disease

The main purpose of adjusting of cultural practices is to seed healthy seeds in healthy soil and to obtain a healthy crop stand.

1. Crop rotation

In plant pathology, crop rotation means using plant to manage plant pathogens. If a particular crop is grown continuously on the same piece of land, the crop gets disease easily, because pathogens survive due to regular presence of susceptible host. Regular crop rotation can control the diseases in the following ways.

- The physical, chemical and biological effects of different crops cause unfavorable soil environment to the pathogens.

- The survival ability of pathogen in soil is limited. By changing the crop every year, their population can be reduced by starvation due to lack of host.
- Better growth of crop plants due to better nutrient availability also helps in avoiding disease.

Most of the soil-borne diseases can be reduced by adopting proper crop rotation. Its success depends upon proper selection of crops in the sequence and knowledge of the survival of the pathogen. The crops between two susceptible host crops should be resistant to the particular pathogen. Along with this the mode of survival and longevity of pathogen in soil should also be know. For example, if the pathogen can survive in the soil for two years, the interval between susceptible crops should be more than two years. Pigeon pea wilt causing fungus infects only pigeon pea crop but after harvesting the crop the pathogen remains in the dead roots of the plant. So there should be a gap of at least one year after growing pigeon pea in the field.

2. Fallowing

Fallowing, is the mode of preparing land, by ploughing it a considerable time before it is ploughed for seed. It is normally adopted in plant disease management for killing pathogens persisting in soil or in crop residues. For fallowing the field should remain weed free. Though fallowing is an alternative method for reducing pathogen population it is often resorted to because of the economic consideration. Fallowing is of three types: (a) dry fallowing, (b) wet fallowing and (c) flood fallowing.

Wet fallowing

In wet fallowing frequent irrigation is given during the fallow period. It is usually practiced for some weeks. The main aim is to make the pathogen germinate in the soil which later dies due to lack of host plant. Wet fallowing reduced the pathogen population especially of sclerotia which retains viability in dry conditions for several years. It is also partly successful in reducing the population of *Pythium* and *Alternaria* .

Dry fallowing

Dry fallowing is generally used where other methods of dis-infestation of soil pathogens are not economical. In this method the field is kept as such for a period of one season to kill the pathogen by starvation.

Flood fallowing

In flood fallowing the land is kept submerged and the pathogens die due to lack of oxygen. Rotting of plant debris also releases materials toxic to pathogens.

3. Soil Solarization

Soil solarization is an advanced field technology for the management of soil borne pathogens. This non chemical management procedure has been adopted by farmers in several parts of the world. It is based on the trapping solar irradiation by tightly covering the soil, usually with transparent polythene sheets. This results in significant increases (10-15°C above normal temperature) of soil, temperature up to the point where most pathogens are vulnerable to heat effects. Soil solarization offers multiple disease control. It controls parasitic diseases, soil borne pathogens, weeds and improves soil suppresiveness and fertility. Major parasitic fungi and diseases managed successfully include damping off, root rots, stem rots, fruit rots, wilts and blight. Among the nematodes *Ditylenchus dipsci, Globodera rostochiensis, Heterodera* spp. and *Meloidogyne* spp. have been managed successfully. Bacterial canker of tomato successfully controlled by solarization for 1-2 months.

4. Mixed cropping

Mixed cropping is growing of two or more crops simultaneously on the same piece of land. It reduces the economic loss from diseases. The reduction in disease incidence in a mixed crop can be attributed to following causes.

- Due to reduced number of host plants there is sufficient spacing between them and chances of contact between foliage or roots of diseased and healthy plants are greatly reduced.
- The roots of non host plants may act as a physical barrier obstructing the movement of pathogen in soil. They may also release toxic substances in their root exudates which suppress the growth of pathogens attacking the main crop. HCN in root exudates of sorghum is toxic to *Fusarium udum* attacking pigeon pea in the mixture.
- Due to reduced number of host pants in a mixed crop the susceptible area for an air borne foliar pathogen is decreased. Therefore, there is less primary infection and less production of secondary inoculums for spread of the disease. This slow down the rate of disease control.
- By proper selection of crops for the mixture, soil environment can also be changed to one that is not favorable for the pathogen. Control of root rot of cotton by growing cotton with moth is an example.
- The soil borne pathogens are not uniformly distributed in the field soil. Generally they are randomly present as dormant structures. Activation of these dormant structures is often dependent on contact with host roots. The chances of which are highly reduced in mixed crop due to spacing between plants.

5. Adjustment of sowing dates:

The sowing time is adjusted in such a way that it reduces the infection period of a pathogen to meet the susceptible stage of the host plant to the minimum. It can be achieved by changing the date of sowing so that the susceptible stage of plant growth does not coincide with the environments highly favorable for the pathogen. Bunt of winter wheat can be controlled by either planting before mid September or after mid October. Early planting of potatoes enables the crop to reach tuberization stage before the insect viz. aphid, reaches it peak in the months of January.

But this sowing time adjustment also has some disadvantages. For example, late sown pea can reduce the extent of early root rot and wilt, but during pod formation stage in late sown pea, powdery mildew and rust will affect the crop. Therefore the farmer has to select the planting date according to the importance of a particular disease in his locality.

6. Sowing depth

Sowing depth can also be adjusted with due regard for soil type and moisture to shorten the period of emergence and to reduce the incidence of damping off disease in many crops. In heavy soil, seed should be placed shallow as compared to light soils. Similarly, in dry soil the seed should be placed deeper in the moist zone, while if water is available irrigate the field before sowing of the a few centimeters and then sow the seeds.

7. Spacing

Of late, the production technology emphasizes on high plant population for getting high yields. But it facilitates luxuriant plant growth, which can cause disease. Luxuriant vegetative growth due to high fertilizer dose, himidity and solar radiation combined with lack of aeration and light to plants, invites pathgen and favours their rapid growth. Damping off ,late blight of potato and mildew of grape vines are some of the diseases which spread fast in close spaced plantings.

But there are also examples where dense sowing help in disease reduction. For example, virus of leaf disease of tomato transmitted by white fly is less in crowded planting than in wide spaced planting. The same is true for cucumber mosaic and groundnut rosette transmitted aphids. Incidence of fungal disease of brown rot of soybean and wilt in cotton is reduced in close sown crop.

8. Plant nutrient management

The relationship between pathogen and crop can be affected by the application of nutrients, viz. nitrogen, phosphorus and potassium. Field applied with potassium fertilizer is less affected by cereal rusts as compared to the fields where no potash is applied. Deficiency of calcium promotes wilt disease in tomato. Similarly, downy mildew infects maize crop due to lack of zone in the soil. The heavy dose of fertilizer also has some disadvantage. For example, late blight of potato in severe due to thick canopy resulting from high nutrition. In such cases, either reduce nitrogen dose or adjust plant spacing. In many crops, nitrogen dose is reduced if crop is already infected by any disease because nitrogen makes plant succulent.

9. Irrigation

The amount of water given in an irrigation should be enough only to wet the soil so that the roots easily get water. If water is in excess, it directly affects the activities of pathogen. As examples, wet soil favours club root of crucifers, silver scurf of potatoes and Cercosporella on wheat, while dry soil increases severity of white mold of onion, common scab of potato anf Fusarium diseases of cereals. Damping off diseases caused by Pythium spp. can be decreased by maintaining a dry soil surfacc.Thc charcoal rot fungus *Macrophomina phaseolina* attacks potato when there is a water stress. So by irrigating the field stress is removed and the disease is suppressed.

Sprinkler irrigation increases diseases owning to enhanced leaf wetness and dispersal of propagules of the pathogens by water splashes as in the case of rain.At the same time, it ahs some advantages also such as washing off of inoculums from the leaf surface.

C. Sanitation

Field and plant sanitation is a main part of disease control through cultural practices. This step is essential even if disease or pathogen free seed or propagating material has been used and other recommended cultural practices have been followed. The inoculums present on few plants in the field may nullify in soil or on the plant and in due course of time may be sufficient to nullify the effect of other cultural practices. Therefore, plants bearing such pathogens or plant debris introducing the inoculums in the soil should be removed as early as feasible. For instance, wilt disease pathogen of banana remains in dead roots, rhizomes and upper portions of the plant. When these plant remains are removed there is rapid decline in the population of the pathogen in the soil. Similarly, the wilt of cotton and arhar and root rot of bean are also reduced to some extent by removal of diseased plant debris.

1. Removal of crop debris

The plant stubbles and roots, left in the field form most of the crop debris. The infected crop debris not only harbours pathogen but also provides media for their growth. The fungus of downy mildew of pea, jowar, bajara and maize, powdery mildew of pea and cereals are some of the diseases which remain in crop debris after harvesting the diseases crop. Destruction of crop debris by burning immediately after harvest reduces the amount of innoculum surviving through debris.

Deep ploughing during hot summer (after rabi crop) burries the debris to such depth where pathogen is destroyed easily. Turning of soil also exposes the pathogen present in the deeper zone, to hot temperature during day time and kills them. Letting the field fallow for some time also serves this purpose as pathogen die to starvation.

2. Rouging

Rouging means removal of unwanted crop plants. The removal of diseased plant is an effective measure in reducing the spread of many diseases. It is very effective against virus diseases of filed crops. Rouging not only checks the spread but also reduces the survival of pathogen. In the production of virus free potato tubers for seed and for the control of virus in soybean and other pulse crops, rouging is an effective control. But in large sized fields it becomes difficult to locate all the diseased plants and uproot them.

3. Removal of diseased parts of plant

In trees and vines, sometimes only a small part is affected by the disease. Powdery mildew of grapevine, apple scab, leaf curl of peach, fire blight of apple and pears are such infections which can be recognized and the infected parts can be removed by pruning with care. Pruning is always carried out after harvest and when the tree is reaching dormancy, a stage least susceptible to fresh infections. Pruning also enables the removal of infected fruits and debris for destruction by burning. The fallen leaves, twigs, etc. are removed from the orchard and destroyed. Similarly, during grafting, care should be taken to ensure that neither stock nor scion is affected by an diseases.

4. Crop free period and Crop free zone

The pathogen attacking crops of secondary importance and having a narrow host range can be controlled by maintaining a crop free period of definite duration. When the growers in an area agree not to grow the crops susceptible to the pathogen for a definite period, depending on longevity of the pathogen without its host , the pathogen is automatically starved out. Similarly, when the host crop is not grown in a zone surrounding the infested area, spread of the disease is checked.

On this basis , for control of bunchy top of banana, it has been suggested that a crop free belt around the area affected by the disease checks it spread provided disease planting material is also quarantined and insect vectors are unable to cross crop free zone. This method is effective for those diseases which are not seed borne and either there is no insect vector or if insect vectors spread then their flight range is limited.

5. Creating barriers by non-host or dead hosts

The spread of majority of diseases from one plant to another in the same field depends on the proximity of healthy roots to infected roots. Growing of other crop in between as in mixed cropping creates barrier by the presence of roots of non-host crops in between.One of the control measure for bacterial wilt of banana and spreading decline of citrus is to destroy the healthy plants around the diseased plants. This checks the movement of pathogen from diseased to healthy plants that are left in the field.

6. Weed management

Weeds are the alternate host of many pathogens. They carry over the pathogen from one season to another and also provide a base from which pathogen is multiplied. For instance, powdery mildew of cucurbits persists on wild cucurbit plant during winter season. Kans grass is an alternate host of sugarcane smut and downy mildew of sugarcane.

7. Adjustment of harvesting time and other practices

The time and method of harvesting is chosen by considering sanitary precautions so that the quality of produce especially fruits and vegetables, does not deteriorate. It also reduces the chances of carrying over the pathogen from the current season to the next. The hill bunt and karnal bunt of wheat, cyst nematode of potato and parasite Orobanche are some of the examples of plant pathogens which are spread in the field during harvesting. Spores of many seed-borne smuts such as karnal bunt of wheat, covered smut of barley and grain smut of sorghum, reach the healthy seeds during harvesting also enables the smut balls, ergot of pearl millet, and ear cockle of wheat to get mixed with the seed lot and contaminate it for next season. To remove these diseases, the following measures should be practiced.

1. Removal of dis eased plants and their affected heads as and when they are noticed.

2. Harvesting under conditions unfavourable to the pathogen; for example, digging out potatoes in dry warm weather reduces the infection of mobile spores called zoospores of late blight can check the bacterial disease transmission up to some extent.

Model Practice Questions

A. Objective Questions

a. Multiple choice Questions

1. Manipulation /or adjustment of crop production techniques for management of plant disease

    (a) Cultural management (b) Physical management

    (c) Biological management (d) Chemical management

2. The disease controls affected by cultural practices are mostly

    (a) Preventive (b) Curative

    (c) Systemic (d) All

3. Cultural practices that help to reduce disease incidence by avoiding the contact between the pathogen inoculum and the plant is

    (a) Date of sowing (b) Deep ploughing during summer

    (c) Depth of sowing (d) All these

4. Actions made to eradicate the disease after it has become established in a region are referred to as

    (a) Exclusion (b) Eradication

    (c) Protection (d) Therapy

5. Roughing is employed to control

    (a) Loose smut of wheat (b) Loose and covered smut of barley

    (c) Wilt of arhar (d) All above

6. Tuber indexing' is a special method to obtain disease free seed materials in

    (a) Potato (b) Tomato

    (c) Brinjal (d) Bhindi

7. pH unfavorable to common scab pathogen of potato

    (a) <5.2 (b) 6.0

    (c) 7.0 (d) >8.0

8. pH unfavorable to club root pathogen of cabbage
   (a) 5.5 (b) 6.0
   (c) 7.0 (d) 4.0
9. The oldest and cheapest method adopted in agriculture for eradication of certain types of pathogens from infested soil
   (a) Crop rotation (b) Mixed cropping
   (c) Companion cropping (d) All
10. Intercropping of sorghum in pigeonpea field reduced the incidence of
    (a) Wilt (b) Phytophthora blight
    (c) Sterility mosaic (d) Collar rot
11. Root exudates of sorghum is toxic to *F. udum*, the pigeonpea wilt fungus due to secretions of chemical
    (a) HCN (b) HCl
    (c) NH_4 (d) CO_2
12. The non-host crops sown with the purpose of making soilborne pathogens waste their infection potential
    (a) Decoy crop (b) Trap crop
    (c) Companion crop (d) Barrier crop
13. Silicon application reduces which disease of rice.
    (a) Blast (b) Bacterial blight
    (c) Sheath blight (d) Sheath rot
14. Removal of alternate host barberry helps to prevent and check the spread of wheat disease
    (a) Black rust (b) Brown rust
    (c) Yellow rust (d) Flag smut
15. Zinc application reduces which disease of rice.
    (a) Blast (b) Bacterial blight
    (c) Sheath blight (d) Khaira

Q. No	Answer	Q. No	Answer
1	(a) Cultural management	9	(a) Crop rotation
2	(a) Preventive	10	(a) Wilt
3	(d) All these	11	(d) Khaira
4	(b) Eradication	12	(a) Decoy crop
5	(a) Loose smut of wheat	13	(a) Blast
6	(a) Potato	14	(a) Black rust
7	(a) <5.2	15	(a) Blast
8	(c) 7.0	16	-

b. True/False

1. Cultural management offer an opportunity to alter the environment,the condition of the host, behavior of the causal agent to achieve economic management of disease.
2. The main purpose of adjusting of cultural practices is to *seed healthy seeds in healthy soil and to obtain a healthy crop stand.*
3. Groundnut blight is controlled by ploughing the soil to a depth of 20 cm.
4. Rapeseed sown in mid to late august is more liable to attack by leaf spot (*Alternaria brassicae*) than late-sown crops.
5. Peas and chickpea sown in october usually suffer heavily from root rot and wilt.
6. Foot rot of ginger is also controlled by following the raised bed system of nursery.
7. Deep planting may cause delay in the emergence of seedlings, which may be vulnerable to pre-emergence damping off.
8. Early and late blight of groundnut are more in dense canopy.
9. Crop rotation is essentially a preventive measure and has its effect mainly on the succeeding crop.
10. Crop rotation with sugarcane or paddy is effective in the control of Panama wilt' of banana.
11. Fodder sorghum can be raised as a trap crop to reduce downy mildew of sorghum.
12. Aluminium strips are used as mulch to protect red peppers against CMV and PVY.
13. Potassium application reduces the disease incidence in many crop diseases probably by increasing phenolics synthesis in plants.
14. Wet fallowing reduces saprophytic survival of *Alternaria solani* on crop debris.
15. Field and plant sanitation is an important method of disease control through cultural practices

Answer

Q. No	Answer	Q. No	Answer
1	True	9	True
2	True	10	True
3	True	11	True
4	True	12	True
5	False	13	True
6	True	14	True
7	True	15	True
8	True	16	-

B. Descriptive Questions

a. Short Answers

1. Write down the role of mixed cropping ind disease management with suitable eaxaples.
2. Write down the role of field and plant sanitation in disease management.
3. How does soil solarization benefit plant health?
4. Write down the basic principles of cultural Practices for disease control.
5. Explain role of wet fallowing in disease management with suitable examples.

b. Long Answers

1. Discuss in details the plant disease management by modification of agricultural practices.
2. Which type of disease can effectively managmed by crop rotation ?
3. How does crop rotation serve as an effective cultural practice in managing plant diseases?
4. Descrive the role of mixed cropping and fallowing in plant disease management.
5. What is cultural management? Write down the procedures for disease management through cultural practices.
6. Give a detail account on use of cultural practices for plant disease management.
7. Describes the role of field and plant sanitation in plant disease management.
8. In what ways can proper plant spacing and plant density influence the development of plant diseases.

9. How plant diseases are influenced by macro and micro nutrients.
10. How does soil management contribute to the prevention and control of plant diseases.

15

Biological Management

Managing plant diseases is necessary to preserve the quantity and quality of food, feed, and fiber that producers worldwide produce. To avoid, lessen, or manage plant diseases, several strategies may be employed. Aside from using effective horticultural and agronomic techniques, growers frequently largely depend on chemical pesticides and fertilizers. The remarkable increases in crop productivity and quality over the past 100 years have been largely attributed to such agricultural inputs. However, fear-mongering by certain opponents of pesticides and environmental degradation from excessive and improper use of agrochemicals have prompted significant shifts in public perceptions toward pesticide usage in agriculture. Political pressure is present to remove the most dangerous chemicals from the market, and there are stringent limits on the use of chemical pesticides today. Furthermore, because of the potential scale at which such applications could need to be made, the proliferation of plant diseases in natural ecosystems may make the successful application of pesticides impossible. As a result, several researchers studying pest management have concentrated on creating substitutes for artificial chemicals in the management of diseases and pests. Biological controls are one type of alternative among them.

Defnition of Biocontrol

Biological control is the reduction of inoculums density or disease producing activities of a pathogen or parasite in its active or dormant state, by one or more organisms accomplished naturally or through manipulation of the environment, host or antagonist, or by mass introduction of one or more antagonists.

Mechanism of Biocontrol

Major mechanism of biocontrol are

1. **Competition:** Competition could involve all kinds of interplay between organisms in which one is favored at the expense of the other. But in strict sense, if we keep antibiosis or even exploitation restricted to their specific mode of action and results, competition has been defined as a more or less active demand in excess of the immediate supply of material or condition on the part of two or more organism.

2. **Antibiosis:** Antibiosis is defined as the condition in which one or more metabolites excreted by an organism have harmful effects on one or more other organism. In such antagonistic relationship species A produces a chemical substance that is harm or inimical to species B without species A deriving any direct benefit. However, the species A may have an indirect benefit in having a better competitive ability, thereby getting an advantage over species B for substrate colonization.
3. **Mycoparasitism:** Mycoparasitism is an act where one fungus parasitizes the other one. The mycoparasitism is of common occurrence and examples can be found among all groups of fungi from chytrids to the higher basidiomycetes. The mycoparasitism includes different kinds of interaction, viz. coiling of hyphae, penetration, production of haustoria and lysis of hyphae.
4. **Antagonism:** Antagonism implies that in any association of two or more species, at least one of the interacting species is harmed due to the activities of one or more of the rest.
5. **Exploitation:** When species A inflicts harm by the direct use of species B for its own benefit, it is exploitation (parasitism and predation). The two terms parasitism and predation have basically same effects, i.e., destruction of the host or prey. In parasitism, some sort of etiological relationship between the parasite and the host is established and the host is not rapidly eliminated. A predator physically eliminates its prey by direct feeding on it without establishing any etiological relationship.
6. **Hypovirulence**: Phenomenon of reduced virulence of a pathogen strain than normal one developed as a result of its infection by ds RNA.
7. **Induction of host resistance**: Plants respond to a variety of chemical stimuli produced by soil- and plant-associated microbes. Such stimuli can either induce or condition plant host defenses through biochemical changes that enhance resistance against subsequent infection by a variety of pathogens.

Some examples of mechanism of biocontrol

S. No	Mechanism	Examples
1	Hyperparasitism / Mycoparasitism	*Trichoderma harzianum* paraitize mycelia of *Rhizoctonia and Sclerotium*
2	Antibiosis	HCN produced by *Pseudomonas fluorescens* Bacilysin produced by *Bacillus subtilis* Trichodermin produced by *Trichoderma*

3	Competition	Exudates/leachates consumption. Siderophore escavenging Physical niche occupation.
4	Induction of host resistance	ISR mediated resistance in tobacco, Aridiopsis Rhizobacteria applied to seeds or roots induce systemic resistance response expressed against pathogens infecting aerial tissues.
5	Hypovirulence	Hypovirulence of fungal pathogens by mycovirus.

Role of Biocontrol

1. **Disease control** :*Trichoderma* is a potential biocontrol agent and used extensively for post harvest disease control. It has been used successfully against various pathogenic fungi belonging to various genera, *viz, Fusarium*, *Phytophthora, Sclerotia.*
2. **Plant growth promoter**: Biocontrol agents solublize phosphates and micronutrients. The application of biocontrol *viz Trichoderma/ Pseudomonas* with plants such as grasses increases the number of deep roots, thereby increasing the plant's ability to resist drought.
3. **Stimulation of plant resistance and plant defense mechanism**: Species of *Trichoderma* or *Pseudomonas* added to the rhizosphere protect plants against numerous classes of pathogens including viral, bacterial and fungal, which points to the induction of resistance mechanisms similar to the hypersensitive response (HR), systemic acquired resistance (SAR), and induced systemic resistance (ISR) in plants.
4. **Transgenic plants**: Introduction of endochitinase gene from *Trichoderma* into plants such as tobacco and potato plants increased their resistance to fungal growth. Selected transgenic lines are highly tolerant to foliar pathogens such as *Alternaria alternata*, *A. solani,* and *Botrytis cinerra* as well as to the soil borne pathogen, *Rhizoctonia* spp.
5. **Bioremediation**: *Trichoderma* strains play an important in the bioremediation of soil that are contaminated with pesticides and herbicides. They have the ability to degrade a wide range of insecticides: organocholorines, organophosphates and carbamates.

Advantages and Disadvantages of biocontrol

Even though it appears as if these biocontrol agents are the cure-all, there are distinct advantages and disadvantages to using them, when compared to traditional chemical controls.

Advantages of biocontrol

- Perform preventive control.
- Low persistence and residual effect.

- Mostly biodegradable and self perpetuating.
- Delayed knock down effect.
- Less resistance prone.
- Less pest resurgence.
- Less harmful on beneficial microorganisms.
- Mostly target specific.
- Waiting period almost nil.
- Costlier but reduced number of applications required.

Disadvantages of biocontrol

- Lack of faith and inconsistent field Performance.
- Poor quality and shelf life.
- Competition with chemical pesticides.
- High budget of production and lesser agribusiness.
- Registration process is expensive and also time- consuming.
- Lack of knowledge, confidence and awareness in end user.
- Inclination towards use of chemical pesticides.
- Non availability of popular literature.
- Mass production of biotic agents limited techniques for indigenous and exotic use.
- Laboratory evaluation of biotic agents and their field efficiency.
- Transfer of technology requires more attention.

The most commonly used biocontrol agents for control of plant pathogens are

1. Trichoderma.
2. Plant Growth Promoting Bacteria (PGPR).

What is *Trichoderma*?

Trichoderma, genus of asexually reproducing fungi, is present in nearly all tropical and temperate soils. The strains of *Trichoderma* spp. are strong opportunistic invaders, fast growing, prolific producers of spores and powerful antibiotic producers. These properties make these fungi ecologically very successful and are the reason for their ubiquitousness. They show a high level of genetic diversity, and can be used to produce a wide range of products of commercial and ecological interest The most common BCAs of the Trichoderma genus are strains of *T. viride*, *T. virens* and *T. harzianum*. Several plant diseases caused by fungi can be potentially controlled by *Trichoderma* species

Importamt plant diseases controlled by *Trichoderma* species.

Name of the Disease	Disease causing organism	Name of the Crop
Collar rot	*Sclerotium rolfsii*	Elephant foot yam
Damping off	*Pythium, Phytopthora, Fusarium*	Chilli, Tomato, Brinjal
Rhizome rot	*Pythium, Phytopthora, Fusarium*	Ginger , onion
Wilt	*Fusarium oxysporum*	Tomato, Brinjal
Sheath blight	*Rhizoctonia solani*	Maize, Rice

General Characteristics

Colonies, at first transparent on media such as cornmeal dextrose agar (CMD) or white on richer media such as potato dextrose agar (PD(a). Mycelium typically not obvious on CMD, conidia typically forming within one week in compact or loose tufts in shades of green or yellow or less frequently white. Yellow pigment may be secreted into the agar, especially on PDA. A characteristic sweet or 'coconut' odor is produced by some species.

Conidiophores are highly branched and thus difficult to define or measure, loosely or compactly tufted, often formed in distinct concentric rings or borne along the scant aerial hyphae. Main branches of the conidiophores produce lateral side branches that may be paired or not, the longest branches distant from the tip and often phialides arising directly from the main axis near the tip. The branches may rebranch, with the secondary branches often paired and longest secondary branches being closest to the main axis. All primary and secondary branches arise at or near 90° with respect to the main axis. The typical *Trichoderma* conidiophores with paired branches assumes a pyramidal aspect.

Phialides are typically enlarged in the middle but may be cylindrical or nearly subglobose. Phialides may be held in whorls, at an angle of 90° with respect to other members of the whorl, or they may be variously penicillate (gliocladium-like). Phialides may be densely clustered on wide main axis (e.g. *T. polysporum*, *T. hamatum*) or they may be solitary (e.g. *T. longibrachiatum*).

Conidia typically appear dry but in some species they may be held in drops of clear green or yellow liquid (e.g. *T. virens*, *T. flavofuscum*). Conidia of most species are ellipsoidal, 3-5 x 2-4 μm. Conidia are typically smooth but tuberculate to finely warted conidia are known in a few species.

Synanamorphs are formed by some species that also have typical *Trichoderma* pustules. Synanamorphs are recognized by their solitary conidiophores that are verticillately branched and that bear conidia in a drop of clear green liquid at the tip of each phialide.

Chlamydospores may be produced by all species, but not all species produce chlamydospores on CMD at 20° C within 10 days. Chlamydospores are typically unicellular subglobose and terminate short hyphae; they may also be formed within hyphal cells. Chlamydospores of some species are multicellular (e.g. *T. stromaticum*).

Teleomorphs of *Trichoderma* are species of the ascomycete genus *Hypocrea* Fr. These are characterized by the formation of fleshy, stromata in shades of light or dark brown, yellow or orange. Typically the stroma is discoidal to pulvinate and limited in extent but stromata of some species are effused, sometimes covering extensive areas. Stromata of some species (Podostroma) are clavate or turbinate. Perithecia are completely immersed. Ascospores are bicellular but disarticulate at the septum early in development into 16 part-ascospores so that the ascus appears to contain 16 ascospores. Ascospores are hyaline or green and typically spinulose. More than 200 species of *Hypocrea* have been described but only few have been grown in pure culture and fewer have been redescribed in modern terms.

Secret of success of *Trichoderma* as BCAs

The success of *Trichoderma* strains as BCAs is due to their

- High reproductive capacity.
- Ability to survive under very unfavorable conditions.
- Efficiency in the utilization of nutrient.
- Capacity to modify the rhizosphere.
- Strong aggressiveness against phyto pathogenic fungi.
- And efficiency in promoting plant growth and defense mechanisms.

Method of Application of *Trichodema*

The biological control practices of the plant pathogens start with the definite principles and practices. There is no hazard to flora, fauna and life and also no disturbance to soil , water and air on account of biological control practices. The following practices are taken up in biological control of the plant diseases.

Seed treatment : Seed treatment with *Trichoderma* has tremendous potential to make the control a great success especially for seed and seedling diseases in vegetables, fruit forest and other plantation crop nurseries . *Trichoderma* seed treatment increased plant stand, reduced seedling mortality and were effective as the chemical fungicides. Generally seed treatment with talc based *Trichoderma* product @ 4gm/kg of seed is recommended for control of root diseases of crop plants.

Soil application: The talc based formulations of *Trichoderma* are used as soil application by mixing in well decomposed compost before application into soil. The quantity required is high and varies from 125-250 kg/ha. It is mixed with, FYM and broadcast on the soil and then incorporated into soil through harrowing. It is used to control *Fusarium* wilt , *Sclerotium* foot rots and *Macrophomina* root rots. Applied at least 2 weeks before sowing of crops.

Furrow application: It is comparatively economical to broadcasting and is followed in nurseries. The quantity required is 130-160 kg/ha. It should be applied in the open furrows and then covered with the soil. Applied 15 days before sowing of the seeds.

Root zone application: This is used in wide spaced crops such as plantation and fruit crops. The formulation is mixed in soil in the root zone upto one kg/ plant.

Wound treatment: This is used to treat pruning wounds of forest and plantation crops. It is done in peach and plum against silver leaf disease.

Pot culture treatment: This treatment is generally applicable in nurseries .Application of bioagents @ 5gm/kg of soil is recommended.

Seedling treatment: The seedling are dispersed in the solution of *Trichoderma* and then they are taken for sowing to control the seedling blight diseases.

Spraying: The liquid suspension prepared by mixing powder and water to get 10^6- 10^8 cfu /ml and sprayed on to the plant surface and soil surface 4g/ liter of water may prepared.

Plant Growth Promoting Rhizobacteria (PGPR)

The rhizosphere bacteria that can colonize the plant roots have been termed as rhizobacteria by Kloepper and Schroth(1978). The rhizobacteria that are strains of *Pseudomonas fluorescens* and *Pseudomonas putida*, have been regarded to have coevolved with their host plants. The term rhizobacteria has been used to accentuate their intimate association with root. These naturaly occurring, non pathogenic , root colonizing bacteria , may be harmful or beneficial for growth of plants are called deleterious rhizobacteria (DRB) and plant growth promoting rhizobacteria (PGPR), respectively. PGPR, fall under genera *Pseudomonas, Bacillus, Arthrobactor, Achromobacter, Citrobactor, Enterobacter* and *Flavobacterium*.The PGPR besides enhancing growth and yields, are also potential biocontrol agents and are usually isolated from suppressive soils. Most of the PGPR are fluorescent pseudomonas (*Pseudomonas fluorescens* and *Pseudomonas putida* but also include non fluorescent Pseudomonas sp., *Bacillus subtilis* and Serratia spp.

Plant growth promoting rhizobacteria are bacteria that colonize plant roots, and in doing so, they promote plant growth and/or reduce disease or insect damage. There has been much research interest in PGPR and there is now an increasing number of PGPR being commercialized for crops. Organic growers may have been promoting these bacteria without knowing it. The addition of compost promote existing PGPR and may introduce additional helpful bacteria to the field. The absence of pesticides and the more complex organic rotations likely promote existing populations of these beneficial bacteria. However, it is also possible to inoculate seeds with bacteria that increase the availability of nutrients, including solubilizing phosphate, potassium, oxidizing sulphur, fixing nitrogen, chelating iron and copper. Phosphorus (P) frequently limits crop growth in organic production. Nitrogen fixing bacteria are miniature of urea factories, turning N_2 gas from the atmosphere into plant available amines and ammonium via a specific and unique enzyme they possess called nitrogenase. Although there are many bacteria in the soil that 'cycle' nitrogen from organic material, it is only this small group of specialized nitrogen fixing bacteria that can 'fix' atmospheric nitrogen in the soil. Arbuscular mycorrhizal fungi (AMF) are root symbiotic fungi improving plant stress resistance to abiotic factors such as phosphorus deficiency or deshydratation.

The fourth major plant nutrient after N, P and K is sulphur (S). Although elemental sulphur, gypsum and other sulphur bearing mined minerals are approved for organic production, the sulphur must be transformed (or oxidized) by bacteria into sulphate before it is available for plants. Special groups of microorganisms can make sulphur more available, and do occur naturally in most soils.

One of the most common ways that PGPR improve nutrient uptake for plants is by altering plant hormone levels. This changes root growth and shape by increasing root branching, root mass, root length, and/or the amount of root hairs. This leads to greater root surface area, which in turn, helps it to absorb more nutrients.

Ways that PGPR promote plant growth

- Increasing nitrogen fixation in legumes.
- Promoting free-living nitrogen-fixing bacteria.
- Increasing supply of other nutrients, such as phosphorus, sulphur, iron and copper.
- Producing plant hormones.
- Enhancing other beneficial bacteria or fungi.
- Controlling fungal and bacterial diseases.
- Controlling insect pests.

Disease control

PGPR have attracted much attention in their role in reducing plant diseases. Although the full potential has not been reached yet, the work to date is very promising and may offer organic growers some of their first effective control of serious plant diseases. Some PGPR, especially if they are inoculated on the seed before planting, are able to establish themselves on the crop roots. They use scarce resources, and thereby prevent or limit the growth of pathogenic microorganisms. Even if nutrients are not limiting, the establishment of benign or beneficial organisms on the roots limits the chance that a pathogenic organism that arrives later will find space to become established. Numerous rhizosphere organisms are capable of producing compounds that are toxic to pathogens like HCN.

Application of PGPRs

Effectiveness of PGPRs does not depend only on suitable PGPRs strains but also on suitable methods and strategies for introducing and maintaining the organisms in crops.Most of the PGPRs strains arre usually applied as:

- Soil application
- Seed coating
- Foliar spray

Soil application: The granule formulation of the PGPR strain has been developed specially for the soil application. Sometimes it can be placed near the root zone along the seedlings during transplanting.

Seed coating: The application of PGPR strain is quite convenient, as little amount of inoculums is required to disperse it along the seed surface. Seed Coating /bacterization is recommended to those PGPR strain, which have sufficient rhizosphere competence so that they may proliferate easily in rhizosphere , increased to sufficient number to express the biocontrol and growth promoting potentiality. In general the agents like Pseudomonas or Bacillus are applied through seed bacterization. Seed treatment may be given as dry seed treatment, wet seed treatment and slurry seed treatement.

Foliar application: The foliar application of PGPR strain is comparatively less common as compared to seed or soil application. However, for the biocontrol of certain aerial plant pathogens the wet formulation is suspended and applied through sprayng in case of bocontrol of bacterial blight of rice the spray method of Pseudomonas was found to reduce the disease intensity.

Precaution

- Formulation of PGPR should be purchased from an authorized / recommended company shop or retailer. The date of manufacturing and expiry of utilization must be verified before delivery.
- During storage packets should not be exposed to direct sunlight and should also not be stored with chemical fertilizers and pesticides.
- Formulation should be stored in cool, and dry place.
- The entire contents of the pack should be used at one time.

Biopesticides

Defnition

Many biologically based products are currently available, and these products are often referred to as "biorationals" or "biopesticides". Biorational is an undefined term used in broad reference to any biologically based product used in agriculture that includes fertilizers, pesticides, herbicides, plant growth regulators, and various other products. A biopesticides is defined by the U.S. Environmental Protection Agency (EPA) as a pesticide derived from natural materials.

FAO Definition

"A compound that kills organisms by virtue of specific biological effects rather than as a broader chemical poison. Biocontrol agents actively seek the pest. The rationale behind replacing conventional pesticides with biopesticides is that the latter are more likely to be selective and biodegradable."

Classification of Biopesticides

Biopesticides fall into three major classes

- **Microbial pesticides:** contains microorganism as the main active ingredients that function as biological control agents, affecting the pathogen directly or indirectly through the compounds they produce or by stimulating specific plant responses. It consist of bacteria, entomopathogenic fungi or viruses (and sometimes includes the metabolites that bacteria or fungi produce). Entomopathogenic nematodes are also often classed as microbial pesticides, even though they are multi-cellular.
- **Biochemical pesticides** are naturally occurring substances that control pests by non toxic mechanisms. Substances that control diseases in this category include potassium bicarbonate, hydrogen dioxide, phosphorus acids, plant extracts, and botanicals

- **Plant incorporated protectants (PIPs):** are least common type of biopesticide. These are pesticidal substances produced by plants that contains genetic material added to the plant of ten through genetic engineering.(e.g GM crops).

Difference between biopesticde and chemical pesticide

Biopesticides	Chemical pesticides
These do not harm non target species	Nontarget species are also harmed
They do not pollute the environment	Cause pollution; sometimes serious
No harmful residues remain in food, fodder and fibers	Harmful residues may often remain in food, fodder and fibers
Relatively cheaper	Relatively costlier
Insects are expected not to develop resistance to biopesticides	Insects may become resistant, e.g., Heliothis has become resistant to most insecticides
Since they are highly specific, correct identification of the pest is essential	It is often not critical
High specificity may often make the use of two or more biopesticides necessary	Often not required
Performance may be variable due to the influence of biotic and abiotic factors of the environment	This is not often the case

Benefits of biopesticides

- The ability to provide alternative modes of action to traditional products which makes them a critical component in most IPM programs.
- Registration in less time than conventional chemical products because biopesticides exhibit minimal impact on the environment and humans.
- The ability to extend the life of conventional chemicals by providing resistance management benefits in agricultural programs.
- Exemption from tolerances, such as reduced preharvest restrictions and application in environmentally sensitive areas, which permits biopesticides that have no Maximum Residue Levels (MRLs) to be used on crops intended for export and in urban settings.
- A high degree of worker safety and the shortest reentry intervals allowed by law.
- Value-added benefits, such as improved plant health, yields and quality and an increase in beneficials, in both traditional and organic cultivation programs.

Biopesticides can be used in almost any crop production program because of they offer unique modes of action and have low impact on the environment and human health. They are especially suited for use in:

- Rotation with chemicals in traditional programs to manage for pesticide resistance.
- Certified organic production systems.
- Grower programs where pesticide residue management is important for harvest management and/or export markets.
- Crops with intensive labor demands to gain maximum flexibility in managing work crews.

Disadvantages

- High specificity, which will require an exact identification of the pest/pathogen and may require multiple pesticides to be used.
- Often slow speed of action (thus making them unsuitable if a pest outbreak is an immediate threat to a crop).
- Often variable efficacy due to the influences of various biotic and abiotic factors (Since biopesticides are usually living organisms, which bring about pest/pathogen control by multiplying within the target insect pest/pathogen).
- Living organisms evolve and increases their resistance to biological, chemical, physical or any other form of control. Unless the target population is completely exterminated or is rendered incapable of reproduction, the surviving population will inevitably acquire a tolerance of whatever pressures are brought to bear- this result in an evolutionary arms race.

Some commercially available biocontrol products/biopesticdes to control plant diseases

Product/Trade Name	Species/strain of *Trichoderma*	Agency/Company
Ecofit	*Trichoderma viride*	*Fusarium, Rhizoctonia, Pythium, Phytophthora,Nectria*
Trichogourd	*Trichoderma viride*	*Fusarium, Rhizoctonia, Pythium, Phytophthora,Nectria*
Defense SF	*Trichoderma viride*	*Fusarium, Rhizoctonia, Pythium, Phytophthora,Nectria*
Tricho-X	*Trichoderma viride*	*Fusarium, Rhizoctonia, Pythium, Phytophthora,Nectria*
Biogourd	*Trichoderma viride*	*Fusarium, Rhizoctonia, Pythium, Phytophthora,Nectria*

Product/Trade Name	**Species/strain of *Trichoderma***	**Agency/Company**
Top shield ,Root shield	*Trichoderma harzianum T-22*	*Fusarium, Rhizoctonia, Pythium*
F-Stop	*Trichoderma harzianum*	*Rhizoctonia, Pythium*
Trichodex	*Trichoderma harzianum strain T-39*	*Colletotrichum, Monilinia, Plamopara , Rhizopus, Sclerotinia*
Bioderma	*Trichoderma viride+ Trichoderma harzianum*	*Fusarium, Botryosphaeria, Fusarium*
Ecoderma	*Trichoderma viride+ Trichoderma harzianum*	*Rhizoctonia, Pythium, Phytophthora*
Binap- T&W	*Trichoderma harzianum+ Trichoderma polysporum*	Wood decay fungi
Gilogard and Soil guard	*Trichoderma virens*	*Rhizoctonia, Pythium*
AQ 10 biofungicide	*Ampelomyces quisqualis*	Powdery mildew
Biotrox C	*Fusarium oxysporum* (non pathogenic)	*Fusarium oxysporum*
Fusaclean	*Fusarium oxysporum* (non pathogenic)	*Fusarium oxysporum*
Contans WG, Intercept WG	*Coniothyrium minitans*	*Sclerotinia sclerotiorum Sclerotinia minor*
Diptera biocontrol	*Myrothecium verrucaria*	Parasitic nematode
Polygandron	*Pythium oligandrum*	*Pytthium ultimum*
Galltrol	*Agrobacterium radiobactor* strain 84	*Agrobacterium tumefaciens*
Companion	*Bacillus subtilis strain GB03*	Pythium, Phytophthora,Fusarium, Rhizoctonia
Histick N/T	*Bacillus subtilis Str.MB 1600*	Fusarium, Rhizoctonia, and Aspergillus
Kodiak	*Bacillus subtilis strain GB03*	Fusarium, Rhizoctonia, and Alternaria
Deny	*Burkholderia cepacia*	Fusarium, Rhizoctonia, and several nematode
Biosave10LP, 110	*Pseudomonas syringae*	Botrytis, Mucor, Penicillium
Dagger G	*Pseudomonas fluorescens*	Rhizoctonia, Pythium
Actino-Iron	*Streptomyces lydicus WYEC 108 plus iron*	Pythium, Rhizoctonia, Phytophthora, Verticillium, and Fusarium spp.
Actinovate	*Streptomyces lydicus WYEC 108 plus iron*	Pythium, Rhizoctonia, Phytophthora, Verticillium, and Fusarium spp.
Bio-Save 10 LP Bio-Save 110 Bio-Save 1000	*Pseudomonas syringae strain ESC-10*	Postharvest decay: blue mold, gray mold, mucor rot, and potato dry rot and silver scurf
Cease	*Bacillus subtilis*	Broad spectrum

Model Practice Questions

A. Objective Questions

a. Multiple Choice Questions

1. All kinds of interplay between organisms in which one is favored at the expense of the other

   (a) Competition (b) Hyperparasitism
   (c) Antibiosis (d) Antagonism

2. The condition in which one or more metabolites excreted by an organism have harmful effects on one or more other organism.

   (a) Hyperparasitism (b) Antibiosis
   (c) Antagonism (d) Exploitation

3. An act where one fungus parasitizes the other one

   (a) Hyperparasitism (b) Antibiosis
   (c) Antagonism (d) Exploitation

4. Any association of two or more species, at least one of the interacting species is harmed due to the activities of one or more of the rest.

   (a) Competition (b) Hyperparasitism
   (c) Antibiosis (d) Antagonism

5. When species A inflicts harm by the direct use of species B for its own benefit

   (a) Hyperparasitism (b) Antibiosis
   (c)Antagonism (d) Exploitation

6. Phenomenon of reduced virulence of a pathogen strain than normal one developed as a result of its infection by ds RNA.

   (a) Antagonism b) Exploitation
   (c) Induction of host resistance (d) Hypovirulence

7. Role of biocontrol

   (a) Disease Control (b) Plant Growth Promoter
   (c) Bioremediation (d) All

8. The success of *Trichoderma* strains as BCAs is due to their

   (a) High reproductive capacity. (b) Efficiency in the utilization of nutrient.
   (c) Strong aggressiveness against phyto pathogenic fungi (d) All

9. Treating of seeds with biocontrol agents and then incubating under warm and moist conditions until just prior to emergence of radical is referred as

(a) Seed disinfectants (b) Seed disinfectants

(c) Seed protect ants (d) Seed biopriming

10. Use by of one species of organism to eliminate or control another species of organism---------------------

(a) IDM (b) Biological control

(c) Cultural control (d) Physical control

11. Suppressive soils are known to have high population of

(a) Antagonistic microorganisms (b) Weeds

(c) Propagules of pathogens (d) Nematodes

12. The project directorate of biological control (PDPC) is located at

(a) Hyderabad (b) Mumbai

(c) New Delhi (d) Bengaluru

13. Most widely used biocontrol agent is

(a) *Pseudomonas florescens* (b) *Pseudomonas putida*

(c) *Bacillus subtilis* (d). *Clostridium*

14. Bioproduct containing *Ampelomyces quisqualis* AQ10 is effective against which of the following diseases.

(a) Powdery mildew (b) Downey mildew

(c) Black mildew (d) Late blight

15. An approach to soilborne pest and pathogen management that involves the use of plants primarily from the brassicaceae family in rotation with cash crops is called

(a) Biofumigation (b) Greening

(a) Soil composting (d) Biosuppressing

Q. No	Answer	Q. No	Answer
1	(a) Competition	9	(d) Seed biopriming
2	(b) Antibiosis	10	(b) Biological control
3	(a) Hyperparasitism	11	(a) Antagonistic microorganisms
4	(d) Antagonism	12	(d) Bengaluru
5	(d) Exploitation	13	(a) *Pseudomonas florescens*
6	(d) Hypovirulence	14	(a) Powdery mildew
7	(d) All	15	(a) Biofumigation

b. True/False

1. The PGPR besides enhancing growth and yields, are also potential biocontrol agents.
2. Trichoderma is the most common BCAs used in plant disease management.
3. A predator physically eliminates its prey by direct feeding on it without establishing any etiological relationship.
4. In parasitism, some sort of etiological relationship between the parasite and the host is established and the host is not rapidly eliminated.
5. The application of living organism to control diseases is called biocontrol.
6. Performance of biocontrol may be variable in the field due to the influence of biotic and abiotic factors of the environment.
7. Rhizobacteria applied to seeds or roots induce systemic resistance response expressed against pathogens infecting aerial tissues.
8. The product bioderma is combination of *Trichoderma viride*+ *Trichoderma harzianum.*
9. The biocontrol agent *Ampelomyces quisqualis* is effective against powdery mildew disease.
10. In augumentative application the biocontrol agent is applies at one place at lower population, which later multiplies and spreads to other plant parts and provide protection.
11. Control of potato scab achieved by green manuring is actually biological control.
12. Most fungi and bacteria produce siderophores that sequester the scarce iron .
13. The PGPR inhibits the growth of deleterious rhizobacteria by preventing their iron uptake.
14. The antibiotic phenazine -1-carboxylic acid (PC(a) produced by *P. fluorescens* is responsible for soil suppressiveness.
15. Coating seeds with bacteria before sowing is called seed bacterization.

Q. No	Answer	Q. No	Answer
1	True	9	True
2	True	10	True
3	True	11	True
4	True	12	True
5	True	13	True
6	True	14	True
7	True	15	True
8	True	16	True

B. Descriptive Questions

a. Short answer

1. Describe biopesticides.
2. Describe the Biopesticide Classification System.
3. What distinguishes chemical pesticides from biological pesticides?
4. PGPR's strategies for fostering plant development
5. Describe Trichoderma.

b. Long answer

1. Define biocontrol. Discuss its scope and limitations to control plant pathogens.
2. Write an essay on biological control of plant diseases.
3. What is biological control of plant pathogens? Give some suitable examples where it has been successfully used to control plant diseases.
4. What is a suppressive soil?
5. What are siderophores? How siderophores production by biological control agnets affects plant pathogen.
6. What do you understand by mycoparasitism? Give some suitable examples of mycoparasitism.
7. Differentiate between chemical and biological control.
8. Describe the commercially available fungal biocntorl agents at present along with their trade name.
9. Write down advantage and diasdvantage of biological control.
10. What is biological control?. Discuss various mode of action of biological control agents.
11. Explain the characteristics of an effective biological control agent. How BCAs are screened and developed?

12. Attempts the following :
    a. Suppressive spoils. b. Siderophores c. Antibiosis d. Hypovirulence e. Future of biological control
13. How do you understand by biopesticides? Give name, dose, and disease managmed by three most commonly used biopesticides.'

16

Host Plant Resistance

Definition of Host Plant Resistance (HPR)

Those characters that enable a plant to avoid, tolerate or recover from attacks of pathogens under conditions that would cause greater injury to other plants of the same species.

or

Those heritable characteristics possessed by the plant which influence the ultimate degree of loss done by the disease.

or

The inherent ability of an organism (i.e., the crop plant) to resist or withstand the pathogen is called resistance

Classification of Resistance

Each plant species is affected by hundreds of kinds of pathogen. Frequently a single plant is attacked by hundreds of individuals of a pathogen. Yet, those plants survive which are resistant, adapting a number of mechanisms classified variously.

1. Based on existence

a. Preformed

When the resistance is already present in the plant even I the absence of the pathogen, it is known as preformed, axenic or passive resistance. For instance, mildew resistance in barley variety Nigrete.

b. Induced

When the resistance is not present in the plant in the absence of the pathogen , but with its contact the resistance is induced, it is known as active, apergic or induced resistance. For instance, seedlings of cotton are susceptible to many pests due to absence of gossypol but once infected by *Verticillium,* gossypol is synthesized by induction and seedlings become resistant.

2. Based on type of host response

a. Immune

Immunity is exempt from infection or hundred per cent freedom from disease. No symptom develop. For instance, potato is resistance to karnal bunt.

b. Resistance

Resistance characterizes those situations in which some degree of host pathogen interaction is evoked. Therefore, resistance is partial, that is ,always some symptoms appear contrary to immunity, where no symptoms appear.

c. Tolerance

Tolerance is defined as the inherent or acquired capacity of the host to endure disease. Tolerance means disease tolerance where yield losses are minimum even in the presence of disease. Therefore, tolerance is the capacity of the host genotype to compensate yield losses even when diseases.

3. Based on growth stage of host plant

Various terms such as seedling resistance, post seedling resistance, adult resistance, etc. have regularly been used to reveal the precise stage of the host growth when it shows resistance. For instance, resistance of wheat to leaf rust (*Puccinia recondita)* may be articulated at the "first leaf stage". The term adult plant resistance is used in the logic that a cultivar is susceptible at first leaf stage but at later stages of development it becomes resistant. For instance, adult plant resistance has been reported in wheat varieties having Sr 2 gene for resistance to stem rust.

4. Based on number of genes

a. **Monogenic resistance:** Controlled by single gene.
b. **Oligogenic resistance:** Controlled by few genes.
c. **Polygenic resistance**: Controlled by many genes.
d. **Major gene resistance**: Controlled by one or few major genes (vertical resistance).
e. **Minor gene resistance**: Controlled by many minor genes. The cumulative effect of minor genes is called adult resistance or mature resistance or field resistance. Also called horizontal resistance.

5. Based on mode of inheritance

a. Monogenic (controlled by a single gene)

Monogenic resistance is frequently sufficiently effective to qualify as immunity. It is stable under a broad array of environmental fluctuations, but is generally specific for certain race virulence gene of the pathogen.

b. Polygenic (controlled by several genes).

Polygenic resistance is more sensitive to environmental fluctuations, does not result in immunity, but is more evenly effective against variants of the pathogen.

c. Cytoplasmic

Such resistance is governed by cytoplasmic factors. For instance, all Tms cytoplasm of miaze used in hybrid seed production is susceptible to T race of Southern Corn Blight. Contrary to it , C or S cytoplasm are also male sterile but are resistant to T race of the pathogen.

6. Based on epidemiological terms

a. Vertical resistance

When a plant variety is more resistant to a few races of pathogen than to others, the resistance is called 'vertical' or 'perpendicular'. Vertical resistance reduces the effective amount of initial inoculums from which the epidemic starts. A characteristic of vertical resistance is that the infection rate is as fast in the vertically resistant as the completely susceptible variety after the initial infection has occurred. In other words, the pathogen may mutate and cause severe diseases in the vertically resistant variety. The vertical resistance may break rapidly whenever new races are formed. Vertical resistance is generally controlled by one or few genes thereby the name monogenic or oligogenic.

b. Horizontal resistance

When host resistance is equally effective against all races of a pathogen-it is termed horizontal or 'lateral'. It may operates before or after infection through defense mechanisms which delay or reduce infection, colonization of the plant and/or production of spores by the pathogen. Horizontal resistance is controlled by many genes, there by the name polygenic or multigenic resistance. Each of these genes alone may be rather ineffective against the pathogen and may play a minor role in the total horizontal resistance.

Horizontal resistance is recommended for subsistence agriculture while vertical resistance is for intensive agriculture.

Diverse complementary terms have been in use to illustrate the genetic concept of resistance. They are summarized in Table.

Terms often used to convey genetic concept of resistance

General Resistance	Specific Resistance
Horizontal	Vertical
Minor	Major

Polygenic	Monogenic
Race nonspecific	Race specific
Quantitative	Qualitative
Multiple gene	Multiple allele
Durable	Nondurable
Non hypersensitive	Hypersensitive
Low to moderate	High

7. Based on mechanism of resistance

The various mechanisms of disease resistance are as follows

1. Mechanical

Mechanical or structural resistances are due to external or internal peculiarities of the host plant. The first line of defense is the surface. Thick hairs, cuticle, wax and hairs on plant parts and foliage check the germination and entry of pathogen in the host tissue. The epidermal cells of rice varieties resistant to blast are lignified. Formation of cork layer beyond the infection point of *R solani* in potato , or abscission layer around diseased spot in peach against *Xanthomonas pruni* are the few examples to further check the spread of pathogen.

2. Hypersensitivity

In the large number of cases, immune reaction is due to he hypersensitive reaction of the host. The mechanism is found in case of biotrophic organisms or obligate parasites. Immediately after infection, several host cells surrounding the point of infection die. This leads to death of the pathogen or at least prevents its spore production.

3. Nutritional

The reduction in growth and in spore production is generally supposed to be due to an unfavorable physiological conditions within the host. Most likely, a resistant host does not fulfill the nutritional requirements of the pathogen and thereby limits its growth and reproduction.

8. Based on population/Line concept

Pureline resistance: Exhibited by lines which are phenotypically and genetically similar.

Multiline resistance: Exhibited by lines which are phenotypically similar but genotypically dissimilar.

9. Miscellaneous categories

Cross resistance: Variety with resistance incorporated against a major disease, confers resistance to minor disease.

Multiple resistance: Resistance incorporated in a variety against different environmental stresses like insects, diseases, nematodes, heat, drought, cold, etc.

10. Based on evolutionary concept

Sympatric resistance: Acquired by coevolution of plant and disease (gene for gene). Governed by major genes.

Allopatric resistance: Not by co-evolution of plant and disease.

Governed by many genes

11. Based on Ecological Resistance or Pseudo resistance

Apparent resistance resulting from transitory characters in potentially susceptible host plants due to environmental conditions.

Pseudo resistance may be classified into 3 categories

a. Host evasion

Host may pass through the most susceptible stage quickly or at a time when insects are less or evade injury by early maturing. This pertains to the whole population of host plant.

b. Induced Resistance

Increase in resistance temporarily as a result of some changed conditions of plants or environment such as change in the amount of water or nutrient status of soil.

c. Escape

Absence of infestation or injury to host plant due to transitory process like incomplete infestation. This pertains to few individuals of host.

Following situations may explain the disease escape

- Early maturing or short duration variety may escape serious disease attack (wheat rust and potato late blight).
- Rapid germination of seed and growth of seedling may escape attack by damping off pathogens.
- Perceptive growth stage of host may not coincide with conducive condition for disease development(*Botrytis* and *Alternaria* are more severe on old senescing plants)
- Plant may escape owing to patchy distribution of soil inoculums.
- Environmental conditions (temperature, humidity, wind and rain) play crucial role in escape of disease. Good planning and adjustment of cultural practices may help to lessen the diseases.

Difference between vertical and horizontal resistance

Factor	Complete Resistance	Partial resistance
Synonyms	Monogenic inheritance Race specific resistance Major gene resistance Juvenile plant resistance Vertical resistance	Polygenic inheritance Non-race specific Minor gene resistance Adult plant resistance Field resistance Rate-reducing resistance Horizontal resistance
Genetic control	One or few genes	Few to many genes
Expression by host	Usually all growth stages	Increases with plant development; lower expression by seedlings
Mechanism	Limits initial infection; none to low symptom development and pathogen reproduction	Slow progress of infection, colonization, lesion development and pathogen reproduction – resulting in slowed disease progress
Efficiency	Highly efficient to avirulent races; high degree of failure against virulent races	Some degree of symptom severity and pathogen reproduction, but similar reaction to all races of pathogen
Primary inoculum	Primary inoculum has little effect	Effectiveness declines as primary inoculum increases; most true for monocyclic diseases
Secondary inoculum	Not a factor because primary inoculum failed to form	Slowed pathogen reproduction; plus fewer successful infections
Environment	Usually stable across range of environments	Effectiveness declines as environment favors pathogen or predisposes host
Pathogen virulence	Exerts strong selection pressure on pathogen population; emergence of new races	Exerts weak selection pressure on pathogen population; slows emergence of new races
Other control tactics	Limited response to additional control tactics	Enhance effectiveness of other control tactics

Resistance Breeding

Resistance breeding differs from breeding for any other traits (quantitative or qualitative), in that one will have to consider the biology of the pest over and above the breeding system of crop plants and the types and genetics of resistance. The use of disease resistant crop plants is an environmentally favourable method of controlling disease but the process of breeding for disease resistance is subject to several constraints among them is the variability of pathogens in relation to host resistance race specific and race non specific resistance. The use of specific resistance demands the identification and use of strong genes against which the stabilizing selection operates.

There are various ways in which strong gene can be used.

- Singly
- Deployment
- In combination
- Multiline

a. Use of Single Resistance Gene

Here the single gene is used one at a time. This strategy results in homogeneity of the crop, which imposes strong selectional pressure on pathogen population. As a consequence there is a development of a race which can over come this resistance and thus there starts a boom –bust cycle. The use of single R-gene is thus risky and its use has been questioned on the ground of its failure to provide permanent resistance.

b. Gene Deployment

This involves distribution of varieties with different resistance genes in space (spatial gene deployment) and in time (temporal gene deployment). The geographical or temporal deployment of varieties with different R. gene causes disruptive selection. Different R gene can be sued in different seasons where more than one crop is taken per year. Gene deployment in space would be most effective against pathogens/ parasite that migrate over long distance and cycling against those that do not. Thus, by adopting such strategy, the stabilizing could be switched on and off and directional selection is thus under human control. Here R- gene could be stored and used again at later date i.e. recycling of R- gene can be done. This sequential pattern involves regular control of disease through changes from R-gene to another. The gene deployment strategy has been used for controlling many plant diseases such as bacterial blight of rice, rusts of wheat, crown rust of oat, leaf rust of barley, rust of bean etc.

c. Pyramiding of genes

When two or more known resistance genes are introduced into a single variety it is called pyramiding or stacking of gene. The aim here is to increase the strength of vertical resistance by way of combining to such a point that the matching pathogen genotype lacks ability to overcome the combined resistance. It increases the longevity of resistance due to low probability of mutation to multiple virulence. Considering mutation rates, 4 or 5 genes for resistance might provide stable resistance for centuries. This has been successfully attempted in a number of crops against different diseases *viz,* rusts of wheat, bacterial leaf blight of rice, blast of rice, rust of bean, powdery mildew of pea etc.Pyramiding of genes for susceptible resistance may act in complementary or additive fashion and thus enhance the level of resistance shown by one particular gene separately.

Thus this approach is superior to gene deployment or multilines. However, the problems in developing a variety with combined resistances are as follows:

- Many of the desired resistance genes are allelic or closely linked and so cannot be easily combined.
- As the sources of different resistance, genes will be different host plants, which may create breeding problems, or the isolated advanced line may have undesirable characters linked with resistance gene.
- The development and cultivation of varieties with multi genes for resistances may lead to the development of super race sooner.

d. Multilines

The introduction of genetic variability in host population through development of multiline can reduce the fitness of the pathogens and thus can break the boom and bust cycle. Multiline varieties are mixtures of several purelines of similar height , flowering and maturity dates, seed color and agronomic characteristic, each of which has a different gene for resistance to athe given disease. The idea of multiline varieties was put forward by Jenson in 1952 for use in cereals. Disease control in multilines can be due to the following reasons:

- Interception of spore by resistant plant called barrier effect.
- Reduction in density of susceptible host variety and the consequent spore production and transmission.
- Induced resistance (due to the non virulent pathogen biotype or cross protection)
- Competitive inhibition
- Modification of micro climate due to different plant types.

Multiline variety appears to be useful approach to control diseases like rusts where new races are continuously produced. In India, three multiline varieties viz., KSML3, MLKS 11 and KML 7406 have been released in wheat.

Boom and Burst Cycle

In varietial improvement programmes, it is easy to incorporate the monogenic vertical resistance genes. But the success of exploiting the monogenic host resistance invariably does not last long. Whenever a single gene-based resistant variety is widely adopted, the impact would be the arrival of new matching pathotypes. These pathotypes soon build up in population to create epidemics and eventually the variety is withdrawn. This phenomenon is generally called " boom and burst". The boom burst cycle can be broken by

- Localized usage of R- gene
- Cycling of R- gene
- Use of polygenic resistance
- Combination of above
- Multigenic resistance
- Multiline variety

Durable resistance

To avoid boom- bust, use of durable resistance is advocated. When a pathogen is not able to overcome the host resistance easily due to fitness reasons, the burst stage is delayed and resistance is noted as durable. This type of resistance remains effective, though the variety is grown over a long period of time. For example, oat variety, Red Rust Proof is still resistant against crown rust even after a hundred years. Wheat varieties, Thatcher and Lee have withstood stem rust for 55 and 30 years, respectively. Cappelle Desprez expresses at adult stage, a moderate resistance to yellow rust and this has been maintained for the last 20 years. Two of the genes like Lr34 for resistance of leaf rust and Sr2 for resistance to stem rust have been recognized for durability. Wheat cultivars such as HD2189, HP1102, DL153-2, DL803-3 and DL802-2, which possess Lr34 with other gene combinations have a good degree of resistance and had become popular with growers.

Vertifolia effect

In the boom and bust cycle, there is a special kind of host erosion of horizontal resistance when Vander plank (1963) has named the vertifolia effect, after the potato cultivar vertifolia which was bred for vertical resistance to blight and which proved exceptionally susceptible when the vertical resistance breakdown. The process of neglecting of losing horizontal resistance in the course of breeding for vertical resistance has been termed as 'vertifolia effect' .This failure occurs because of two reasons:

- The level of horizontal resistance in the varieties carrying oligogenes for resistance is usually low.
- The pathogen is able to evolve the virulent pathotype.

Pre-emptive breeding

Pre-emptive or anticipatory breeding for resistance is breeding for resistance to future patho types. Its success depends n the ability of the breeder to predict the likely pathogen phenotypes (pathotypes) that will be important at some future time. Because durability of resistance can not be assumed, resistance breeding strategies are usually supported with the maintenance of genetic diversity to provide buffering against extreme crop losses in the event of significant pathogenic changes.

Breeding methods for disease resistance

The methods of breeding varieties resistant to diseases do not differ greatly from those adopted for other characters. The following methods are used:

1. Introduction,
2. Selection,
3. Hybridization followed by selection,
4. Back cross method,
5. Induced mutagenesis,
6. Development of multilines and
7. Tissue culture techniques

1. Introduction

It is a very simple, quick and inexpensive method of obtaining resistant varieties. Varieties resistant to a particular disease somewhere else may be thoroughly tested in the regions in which they are proposed to be introduced. Their yield performance and disease resistance should be confirmed by large scale cultivation. Introductions have served as a useful method of disease control.

Resistance variety introduced in India from other countries

Name of Crop	**Name of Variety**	**Introduced from**	**Introduced in**	**Remarks**
Wheat	Ridley	Australia	India	Rust resistance
wheat	Kalyan Sona and Sonalika	CIMMYT, Mexico	India	Rust resistance
Rice	Manila	Philippines,	Karnataka	Tolerance to blast, bacterial leaf blight and sheath blight.
Rice	Intan,	Indonesia	Karnataka	Resistant to blast
Rice	Munal	U.S.A.	West Bengal	Tolerant to blast, bacterial leaf blight and leaf folder
Sugarcane	Co.475		Mumbai	Conquered red rot but brought in leaf rust and whip smut

2. Selection

Selection of resistant plants from a commercial variety is the cheapest and quickest method of developing a resistant variety. This is better method than introduction and has more chances of success in obtaining disease-resistant plants. The work of selection is carried out either in the naturally infected fields under field conditions or under artificially inoculated conditions. The resistance in such individuals will occur in nature by mutation. To ensure the resistant character of a plant, large population of crop plant may be exposed to the attack of pathogen under artificial conditions and the non-infected plants may be chosen. Sugandha of Bihar is a selection from Basmati rice of Orissa tolerant to bacterial leaf blight. Rice varieties Sudha (Bihar), Patel 85 (Madhya Pradesh), Janaki (Bihar), Sabita, Nalini (West Bengal), Improved White Ponni (Tamil Nadu), Ambika (Maharashtr(a), are some of rice selections resistant to one or more diseases. Kufri Red, a potato selection from Darjeeling Red Round is a disease resistant variety.

3. Hybridization

Hybridization is the most common method of breeding for disease resistance, Hybridization serves the following two chief purposes: (1) transfer of disease resistance from an agronomic ally undesirable variety to a susceptible but otherwise desirable variety (by back crossing). And (2) combining disease resistance and some other desirable characters of one variety with the superior characteristics of another variety (by pedigree method).In the back cross method, the new variety is agronomically the same as the susceptible variety, but is disease resistant. In the pedigree method, on the other hand, the new variety is expected to be superior to both the parents in agronomic characteristics and at the same time would be disease resistant.

In both the cases, one parent is selected for disease resistance; it should have a high intensity of resistance to as many races of the pathogen as possible, and the resistance whould be governed by few oligogenes. When the resistant variety is undesirable and agronomically updated, backcross method is the obvious choice. But when the resistant variety is well adapted and has some other desirable features as well, the pedigree method of breeding is preferred. This method is suited for small grains and beans but unsuited to fruits and vegetables.

4. Back cross method

The back cross method is useful in transferring genes for resistance from variety that is undesirable in agronomic characteristics to a susceptible variety, which is widely adapted and is agronomically highly desirable. is widely used to transfer disease resistance from wild species. Interspecific hybridization is made to transfer the gene or genes for resistance to the cultivated species. Resistance to grassy stunt virus from *Oryza nivara* to *O.sativa*, late blight resistance from *Solanum demissum* to cultivated potato, rust resistance from *durum* to *aestivum* wheat are some of the examples involving interspecific hybridization. Depending upon the number of genes governing resistance and the nature of the gene, whether dominant or recessive, the procedure varies. The number of back crosses to the cultivated species may be five to six. Once the back cross progeny resemble the cultivated parent, then they are selfed and segregating progeny screened for disease resistance.

5. Induced mutagenesis

While following mutation breeding for disease resistance, a large number of mutation progeny should be produced and screened under artificial epiphytotic condition to select resistant plants. MCU10 cotton, a resistant variety to bacterial blight was evolved in Tamil Nadu by subjecting seeds of a susceptible variety CO4 to gamma rays followed by rigorous screening and selection. Resistance to Victoria blight (caused by *Helminthosporium victoriae*) in oats was induced by irradiation with X-rays or thermal neutrons; resistant mutants were also isolated spontaneously in low frequencies. Some other cases in induced mutations for disease resistance are as follow; resistance to stripe rust in wheat, crown rust in oats, mildew in barley and leaf spot or tikka in ground nut.

7. Somaclonal variation

Disease resistant somaclonal variants can be obtained in the following ways. First, plants regenerated from cultured cells or their progeny are subjected to disease test and resistant plants are isolated (screening). Secondly, cultured cells are selected for resistance to the toxin or culture filtrate produced by the pathogen and plants are regenerated from the selected cells (Cell selection). In most cases, these plants are also resistant to the disease in question. Cell selection strategy is most likely to be successful in cases where the toxin is involved in disease development. Somaclonal variations for disease resistance are reported in *Zea mays* for *Drechslera maydis* race T-toxin resistance, in *Brassica napus* for resistance/tolerance to *Phoma lingam*, early and late blight resistance in potato, *Pseudomonas* and *Alternaria* resistance in tobacco, besides smut and rust disease resistance in sugarcane.

Testing of Disease Resistance

Disease resistance tests may be carried out in the field or in the glass house. Glass house tests are more reliable since the favourable environment for disease development can be provided more readily in a glass house than in a field.

An optimum humidity and temperature are necessary, though the optimum conditions for one disease may vary significantly from that for another. The common inoculation techniques used for different categories of pathogens are briefly outline below

1. Soil borne pathogens

Diseases *viz.,* damping off, root rot, wilt etc., are produced by fungi present in the soil. Commonly, sick plots are created for testing resistance to such diseases. Sick plots are fields that have a sufficient inoculums load of the pathogen to infect all the susceptible plants of the host population. Sick plot may be produced by adding the remains of diseased plant, or by adding inoculums produced in a laboratory on host seeds, seedlings or on a nutrient medium or by mixing the soil from other sick plots,. The pathogen inoculums may be increased by growing a susceptible variety for one or more years. Glass house tests may be carried out using the soil from a sick plot.

2. Air borne diseases

Diseases like smuts, rusts, blight, mildews, leaf spots etc., are produced by air borne fungal pathogens. Inoculation of such a disease may be done by dusting spores from infected plants onto test plants, spraying a suspension of spores or mycelium , injecting a spore suspension into individual plants or leaves, or, in some cases, by planting rows of a highly susceptible variety, normally called infectior, to produce a large inoculums, which is spread by natural factors, e.g., wind. In the case of wheat rust, infectors are commonly used. Agra Local wheat is the common infector for all the three rusts. In the case of air borne fungi infecting ovary. e.g., loose smut of wheat and barley, spores are introduced in the flowers at the time of anthesis with the help of a forecep or a hypodermic needle.

3. Seed borne diseases

Some diseases are seed borne, e.g., some smuts, bunt etc. Mostly the smut spores are present on the surface of the seed or under the hull. In artificial inoculation of seeds with smut spores, the seeds and spores are thoroughly mixed before planting. In hill bunt of wheat and grain smut of jowar dusting of spores on the seed is enough for inoculation. In smut diseases of barley, oats, etc. usually the seeds are treated with spore suspension under vacuum to facilitate deposition of spores on the seed. In diseases where the pathogen is both soil as well as seed borne mostly soil inoculation is preferred.

4. Insect transmitted diseases

Most of the viral diseases are transmitted either by insects or mechanically. The following procedures are adopted in testing varieties.

a. **Transmission by insect vectors**; Insects which fed on diseased plants are collected and left on healthy plants to continue feeding. Mostly these insects aphids or white fly. The healthy plants are grown in insect proof cages so that unwanted insects do not visit them and the vectors being used do not move out. Obviously, such tests cannot be conducted on a large number of plants under field conditions. The insect vectors must feed on the diseased and healthy plants for the minimum period requirement for becoming infective.

b.Mechanical transmission: The juice from infected plants rubbed on healthy leaves. To facilitate contact with healthy cell sap artificial wounds or scratches are created by rubbing carborundum powder separately or with the infected juice.

Model Practices Questions

A. Objective Questions

a. Multiple choice Questions

1. The decline in the level of horizontal resistance due to continuous breeding for vertical resistance is

   (a) Vertifolia effect (b) Pasteur effect
   (c) Boom and bust cycle (d) Apparent resistance

2. The ability of a plant to sustain the effects of a disease without suffering serious injury or crop loss is

   (a) Resistance (b) Tolerance
   (c) Susceptibility (d) Innate immunity

3. Hypersensitivity is applicable to the plant diseases caused by

   (a) Fungi (b) Bacteria
   (c) Viruses (d) All these

4. When two or more known resistance genes are introduced into a single variety it is called

   (a) Pyramiding of gene (b) Gene deployment
   (c) Vertifolia effect (d) Boom & Bust cycle

5. Strategic use of major gene, by deploying these over space and time to avoid phenomena of boom and bust is called

   (a) Pyramiding of gene. (b) Gene deployment
   (c) Vertifolia effect (d) Boom & Bust cycle

6. When the resistance is already present in the plant even the absence of the pathogen. it is known as

(a) Axenic resistance. (b) Gene deployment

(c) Vertifolia effect (d) Induced resistance

7. The boom burst cycle can be broken by

(a) Localized usage of R- gene (b) Cycling of R- gene

c) Use of polygenic resistance (d) Combination of above

8. The mechanism of disease resistance in plant are

(a) Mechanical (b) Hypersensitivity

c) Nutritional (d) All

9. The gene for gene hypothesis is proposed in disease

(a) Linseed rust (b) Wheat rust

c) Pea rust (d) Barley rust

10. Apparent resistance in crop is achieved by

(a) Early varieties (b) Change date of planting

(c) Change in the site of planting (d) All

11. The inherent ability of an organism (i.e., the crop plant) to resist or withstand the pathogen is called

(a) Resistance (b) Tolerance

(c) Susceptibility (d) Endurance

12. Absence of infestation or injury to host plant due to transitory process like incomplete infestation. This pertains to few individuals of host.

(a) Host evasion (b) Induced Resistance

(c) Disease Escape (d) Boom & Bust cycle

13. Host may pass through the most susceptible stage quickly or at a time when insects are less or evade injury by early maturing. This pertains to the whole population of host plant.

(a) Host evasion (b) Induced Resistance

(c) Disease Escape (d) Boom & Bust cycle

14. Strategic use of major gene, by deploying these over space and time to avoid phenomena of boom and bust is called

(a) Pyramiding of gene. (b) Gene deployment

(c) Vertifolia effect (d) Boom & Bust cycle

15. Major gene, race -specific, seedling, monogenic, differential, specific and pathotype specific resistance is
    (a) Vertical resistance (b) Horizontal resistance
    (c) Apparent resistance (d) Disease Escape
16. Cytoplasmic inheritance is governed by
    (a) Chloroplast DNA (b) Plasmid DNA
    (c) Mitochondrial DNA (d) All of these
17. The plant pathogen regarded as genetic engineer of plant kindgdom is
    (a) *Agrobacterium tumefaciens* (b) *Erwinia amylovora*
    (c) *Neurospora crassa* (d) *Pseudomonas syringae*

18. Non-differential resistance that is uniform, effective against all the races of a pathogen and reduces the rate of disease development is
    (a) Horizontal resistance (b) Vertical resistance
    (c)Apparent resistance (d) Non-host resistance
19. SAR govern by
    (a) Salicylic acid (b) Jasmonic acid
    (c) Ascorbic acid (d) Lactic acid
20. Breeding for resistance to future pathotypes is called
    (a) Introduction (b) Selection
    (c) Hybridization (d) Pre emptive breeding

Q . No	Answer	Q. No	Answer
1	(a) Vertifolia effect	11	(a) Resistance
2	(b) Tolerance	12	(c) Disease Escape
3	(d) All these	13	(a) Host evasion
4	(a) Pyramiding of gene.	14	(b) Gene deployment
5	(b) Gene deployment	15	(c) Viroid
6	(a) Axenic resistance	16	(a) Vertical resistance
7	(d) Combination of above	17	(a) *Agrobacterium tumefaciens*
8	(d) All	18	(a) Horizontal resistance
9	(a) Linseed rust	19	(b) Jasmonic acid
10	(d) All	20	(d) Pre emptive breeding

b.True /False

1. Multiline variety appears to be useful approach to control diseases like rusts where new races are continuously produced.

2. The concept of boom and bust cycle was given by Priestley.
3. The gene for gene hypothesis is proposed by HH Flor.
4. Immunity is exempt from infection or hundred per cent freedom from disease
5. Resistance is partial, that is ,always some symptoms appear.
6. Monogenic resistance is easy to incorporate into plants by breeding.
7. Polygenic resistance is more sensitive to environmental fluctuations.
8. All Tms cytoplasm of maize used in hybrid seed production is susceptible to T race of Southern corn blight.
9. Vertical resistance reduces the effective amount of initial inoculums from which the epidemic starts.
10. Horizontal resistance may delay or reduce infection, colonization of the plant and/or production of spores by the pathogen.
11. Sick plots are created for testing resistance of soil borne diseases.
12. Vertical resistance is also called juvenile plant resistance
13. Horizontal resistance is also called minor gene resistance.
14. Effectiveness of horizontal resistance declines as environment favors pathogen or predisposes host.
15. Vertical resistance exerts strong selection pressure on pathogen population leads to emergence of new races

Answer

Question no	Answer	Question no	Answer
1	True	9	True
2	True	10	True
3	True	11	True
4	True	12	True
5	False	13	True
6	True	14	True
7	True	15	True
8	True	16	-

B. Descriptive Questions

a. Short Answer

1. What is durable resistance? Give five examples of durable resistance.
2. Name two diseases in which the soil moisture determines disease escape.

3. Discuss about i.Gene pyramiding ii.Gene deployment iii. Apparent resistance.
4. Differetiate between horizontal and vertical resistance.
5. Write down the mechanism of disease resistance.
6. What are the disadvantages of growing genetically uniform crops over large areas.
7. Differentiate between disease escape and tolerance.
8. Name four diseases (with their pathogens) that exemplify vertical resistance.
9. Define pathotype, pathodeme, esodemic, exodemic
10. What are Hrp proteins?
11. Write in brief about cross protection

b. Long Answer

1. What is host plant resistance? Classify resistance on the basis of existence, host response and epidemiological competence.
2. Write short notes on a. Boom and Bust cycle b. Vertifolai effect c. Anticipatory breeding d. Multiline.
3. Who first proposed 'gene-for-gene concept'? Name the disease involved with its pathogens.
4. What are resistance genes? Classify them on the basis of their structure and function. Discuss their mechanism of action and evoloution.
5. Give a concise account of genetic resistance in plants.
6. Attempt the following:

a. Boom and bust cycle
b. Genetic recombination in viruses
c. Cytoplasmic resistance
d. Differences between VR and HR
e. Physiological races
f. Avirulence genes.

17

Regulatory Methods Plant Quarantine

Plant Quarantine

The term 'Quarantine' is derived from the Latin word *quarantum,* meaning 40. It refers to the 40 days period of detention of ships from countries with bubonic plague and cholera in the Middle Ages. The first such quarantine was imposed in Venice in 1374.Present quarantine laws now include plants. Plant quarantine , restrict entry of plants, plant products, soil, cultures of living organisms, packing materials, and commodities, as well as their containers and means of conveyance to protect agriculture and the environment from avoidable damage by hazardous organisms.They exclude dangerous organisms while permitting plants and plant products to enter. The term *exclusion* convey this objective more clearly than *plant quarantine.* Exclusion relates to keeping organisms out; plant quarantine relates to keeping plants out.

In strict sense 'Plant Quarantine' refers to the holding of plants in isolation until they are believed to be healthy. Now, broader meaning of the plant quarantine covers all aspects of the regulation of the movement of living plants, living plant parts/plant products between politically defined territories or ecologically distinct parts of them. Intermediate quarantine and post entry quarantine are used respectively to denote the detention of plants in isolation for inspection during or after arrival at their final destination.

The term frequently used in plant quarantine are *hazard, risk*, and *safeguards.*

- **Hazard**: is the danger that a specified pathogen is known or perceived to present to the agriculture of the importing country should the pathogen gain entry on imported items and subsequently become established.
- **Risks**: is the chance that a hazardous organism will enter and become established.
- **Safeguards**: are action taken to reduce the risk of introducing hazardous organisms.

Importance

The importance of plant quarantine has increased because of the increase in exchange of seeds or grains for consumption along with better means of transportation. The international exchange of plants or their parts is practiced widely to improve crops of a country and their genetic base. In addition, shiploads of grains for consumption or large quantities of seeds for direct sowing are imported in many countries. Even minute quantities of soil and plant debris contaminating true seeds can disseminate pathogens.

The entry of a single exotic insect or disease and its establishment in the new environment continues to cause great, national loss till such time it is brought under effective control. In certain cases a country has to spend a few million rupees before success in controlling the introduced insect pest or disease is achieved.

Losses caused by introduced plant diseases

Disease	Host	Country	Introduced From	**Losses Caused**
Bunchy top	Banana	India	Sri Lanka	Rs.4 crores
Wart	Potato	India	Netherlands	2500acres infected
Canker	Citrus	U.S.A	Japan	$ 13 million; 19.5 million trees destroyed
Dutch elm	Elm	U.S.A.	Holland	$ 25 million -$ 50,000 disease million
Powdery mildew	Grapevine	France	U.S.A	80% in wine production
Downy mildew	Grapevine	France	U.S.A	$ 50,000 million
Wart	Potato	India	Netherlands	2500acres infected
Blue mould	Tobacco	Europe	U.K	$ 50 million

Aim of Plant Quarantine

The aim of plant quarantine is to prevent the introduction of dangerous diseases and pests or new races of a pathogen and their spread within the country.

Goal of Plant Quarantine

The goal of regulatory actions are

- To delay or prevent entry of the pathogen along manmade pathways.
- If entry succeeds, to prevent infection.
- If infection succeeds, to prevent establishment of pathogens entering on manmade and natural pathways.
- If established, to minimize or retard spread.

Basic Principles of Plant Quarantine

- The basic principles of plant quarantine is to check the entry and spread of potentially dangerous plant pathogens and insects imported along with the germplasm.

Prerequisites of Plant Quarantine Regulations

In spite of quarantine regulations, plant pathogens have been introduced in different countries. Plant quarantine regulations have certain prerequisites. They must be

- Only pathogens and pest that pose a threat to major crops or forest should be taken into considerations.
- Formulated to control or prevent the pests and not to hinder trade or attainment of other objectives.
- Derived from adequate legislation and operated solely under the law.
- Modified as conditions change or further facts become available.
- Those responsible for quarantine measures should be properly trained and experienced.
- Professional workers and the public must co-operate on an international scale for effective operation of quarantine regulations.

Component of Plant Quarantine

Plant protection and quarantine (PPQ) programs, or the plant health or quarantine services in most countries, usually have three components

1. Exclusion of pathogens and pests of quarantine and economic significance that might unintentionally be moved along manmade pathways when articles are imported, or induction of the risk of introducing such hazardous organisms to an acceptance level.
2. Containment, suppression, and eradication of exotic pathogens and pests recently introduced along natural and manmade pathways.
3. Assistance to exporters of plant products, such as fruits, vegetables, plants, cut flowers, commodities, etc., in meeting the quarantine or exclusion requirements of importing countries and , therefore, based on plant health, biologically facilitating the acceptance of imports.

1. Pest Risk Analysis

Pest risk defines the chances that a pathogen or pest of quarantine significance will enter along a manmade pathway. Risk often is expressed as low, medium or intermediate, and high.

- **Low risk:** means that there is little chance that the pathogen or pest will enter.
- **High risk:** means that chances are high that the pathogen or pest could enter.
- **Acceptable risk:** An acceptable risk level means that the benefits derived after taking risk are high enough to justify taking the risk, with safe guards , in the first place.

The rules and regulations governing seed entry should be based on a matching of risk with entry decisions. If the risk is low, the entry should be liberal; if risk is high, the entry atus should be conservative: and when the risk is unknown, quarantine officer need to be policy of an importing countries might prohibit all plants of high risk and by doing so take no risk, but at the cost of receiving no benefits from crop improvement.

2. Movement of pathogens

Plant pests of quarantine importance can move along with natural and man made pathways, depending upon the life cycle of the organism, the environment through which it moves, and human activities. At the end of the pathway, the establishment of a a pathogen or pest in a new area depend on the level of inoculums or pest carried by seeds, the susceptibility of host crop(s), and the environment. Exchange of germplasm creates the risk of introducing pathogens or pests of quarantine importance. The considerations are two fold; that exotic organisms or more virulent strains of existing ones might be introduced. Quarantine regulations to prevent movement of feaces derived products as a potential source of introduction should be considered. Viable teliospores of *T.caries, T. indica* and *T. controversa* are present in feaces of chickens, grasshoppers and cow. Hence quarantine established to prevent movement of spore contaminated seeds may miss an important avenue of potential introduction by animal and animal product movements.

3. Legal basis of plant quarantine

Quarantines are regulations promulgated by governments to reduce the risk of introducing hazardous pathogens and pests on articles, including seeds from foreign countries. The legal basis of quarantine comprises

- Legislation enacted by national and sometimes state or provincial governments.
- Enabling legislation that directs the Minister of Agriculture to issue necessary rules, orders or directives, or

- Legislation by a regional parliament representing groups of countries such as the EEC or Andean Pact Nations.
- The legal umbrella that covers international plant quarantine matters is the International Plant Protection Covention of 1951 (Rome Certificate). Most countries either are signitories of the Rome Convention or follow its mandates.

4. Requirement for a Quarantine program

- A phytosanitory certificate that attests to the inspection, origin and identification of the seeds.
- A permit requirement for added declaration on the phytosanitory certificate that the mother plants were inspected during the growing season.
- A requirement for treatment at origin.
- The acceptance of a special certification or safe guarding program at origin, such as may be practiced at International Agricultural Research Centers (IARC).
- Inspection and treatment , if necessary ,upon arrival at port of entry; and
- Isolation, special testing, or additional quarantine after entry.

National and International Regulations

- The first plant quarantine law was passed in 1873 in Germany to prohibit importation of plants and plant products from the United States to prevent the introduction of the Colorado potato beetle.
- In 1975, France imposed measures against the American pest.
- In 1877, United Kingdom Destructive Insects Act prevented the introduction and spread of this beetle.
- In 1891, first plant quarantine measure was initiated in the United States by setting up a seaport inspection station at San Pedro, CA.
- In 1912, first U.S. quarantine law was passed.
- In 1909, Federal Plant Quarantine Service was established in Australia.
- In 1914, Destructive Insects and Pest Act was passed in India.
- In 1971, Government of Greece prohibited introduction of rice seeds for sowing infected with *Pyricularia oryzae.*
- In 1980, Phillipine government introduced seed health testing plants of rice for *Pyricularia oryzae* in addition to field inspections for breeder and foundation seeds.

On a global basis, the first International Plant Protection Convention (the Phyllozera Convention) was signed in 1881 with the objective of preventing the spread of severe pests. This convention was amended in 1889,1929 and 1951. The International Plant Protection Convention (IPPC or Rome Convention) under the Food and Agriculture Organization was established to prevent the introduction and spread of diseases and pests through legislation and organizations across international boundaries. This convention provided a model phytosanitary certificate (Rome certificate) to be adopted by member countries. Within this convention, ten regional plant protection organizations have been established on the basis of biogeographical areas

- The European and Mediterranean Plant Protection Organization (EPPO)
- The Inter-African Phytosanitary Council (IAPSC)
- Organismo International Regional de Sanidad Agropecnario OIRSA
- The Plant Protection Committee for, the South East Asia and Pacific region.(SEAPPC).
- Near East Plant Protection Commission (NEPPC)
- Comit'e Interamericano de Protection Agricola. (CIPA)
- The Caribbean Plant Protection Commission (CPPC)
- The North American Plant Protection Organization (NAPPO).
- Organismo Bolivariano de Sanidad Agropecuria (OBSA)
- Association of South East Asian Countries (ASEAN)

The regional organizations are concerned with the co ordination of legislation and regulations within their area, agreement on the quarantine objects, inspection procedures, etc.

Criteria for Determining Organisms for Quarantine Significance

1. General criteria

The following are general criteria considered for an organism of plant quarantine significance:

- The organism does not occur in the country but is known to cause economic damage elsewhere.
- The organism occurs in the country but is not extensively spread in the ecological range of its host in that country; is under a national domestic suppression or eradication programme; has exotic strains of quarantine importance that do not occur in the country; and/or causes economic damage or has a potential to cause such damage on economically important crops.

- The organism is a general pathogens established in the importing country. But government regulations require that commercial growers use pathogen-tested seed stocks so that imported stocks meet domestic standards.

2.Criteria based primarily on Pathogen Characteristics

The criteria are based on the general characteristics of a pathogen.

- Able to survive and move easily in international trade.
- Capable of developing a high population in a short time.
- Difficult to detect by general inspection or field survey.
- Capable of damaging and / or reproducing on many hosts.
- Has a potential for rapid dispersal , especially along manmade pathways.
- Has a potential for significant reduction in the quality and quantity of crop yields.
- Capable of adversely affecting the environment.

Problems in Plant Quarantines

Quarantine serves as a filter against the introduction of dangerous pathogens, however pathogens are still introduced. Probable reasons are that

- Difficult to detect all types of infectious pathogens by conventional methods.
- Methods may not be sensitive enough to detect traces of infection.
- Latent infections may pass undetected under post entry quarantine.
- Destruction of all infected or suspected material and
- Sensitive methods for testing fungicide treated seeds may be lacking.

Organisms of Quarantine Significance

Organisms of quarantine significance may include any pathogen or pest that a government (or intergovernmental organization) considers to pose a threat to the agriculture and environment of the country or region. Such organism generally are exotic to that country or region but may include exotic strains or races of domestic strains.

Plant quarantine methods

There are number of plant quarantine methods which are used individually or jointly to retard or prevent the introduction and establishment of exotic pests and pathogens. The components of plant quarantine activities are:

1. Complete embargoes

This is the most effective measure to exclude specified plants and plant products completely from a country infected or infested with highly destructive diseases or pests or that could be transmitted by the plant or plant products under consideration and against which no effective plant quarantine treatment can be applied or is not available for application. However, in practice it is difficult to achieve because of more and more exchange of diverse genetic material among countries.

2. Partial embargoes

Partial embargoes, applying when a pest or disease of quarantine importance to an importing country is known to occur only in well defined area of the exporting country and an effectively operating internal plant quarantine service exists that is able to contain the pest or disease within this area.

3. Inspection and treatment at point of origin

It involves the inspection and treatment of a given commodity when it originates from a country where pest/disease of quarantine importance to importing country is known to occur.

4. Inspection and certification at point of origin

It involves pre-shipment inspection by the importing country in cooperation with exporting country and certification in accordance with quarantine requirements of importing country.

5. Inspection at the point of entry

It involves inspection of plant material immediately upon arrival at the prescribed port of entry and if necessary subject to treatment before the same related.

6. Utilization of post entry plant quarantine facilities

It involves growing of introduced plant propagating material under isolated or confined conditions.

Plant quarantine organizations in India

The first plant quarantine measure in India dates to 1906, when the danger of introducing the Mexican boll weevil had the Government of India directed that all cotton imported from the New World should only be admitted after fumigation with carbon disulphide. Two categories of regulatory measures are in operation for controlling pests, diseases and weeds:

- Destructive Insects and Pests (DIP) Act of 1914 of Central Government, which regulates the introduction of exotic diseases and pests into the country or their spread from one state or union territory to another.
- The Agricultural Pests and Diseases Acts of various states, which suppress or prevent the spread of diseases and pests in areas within a State or Union Territory.

The legislative measures against crop pests and diseases were initiated under the DIP Act of 1914 which was passed by the then Governor General of India in Council on 3 February 1914. The quarantine regulations are operative through The Destructive Insects and Pests Act, 1914 (which has been revised 8 times from 1930 to 1956 and amended in 1967 and 1992). The provisions of the DIP Act are

- It authorizes the central government to prohibit or regulate the import into India or any part.
- There of or any specific place therein of any article or class of articles.
- It authorizes the officers of the customs at every port to operate, as if the rules under DIP act are made under the Sea Customs Act.
- It authorizes the central government to prohibit or regulate the export from a state or the transport from one state to another state in India of any plants and plant material, diseases or insects, likely to cause infection or infestation. It also authorizes the control of transport and carriage and gives power to prescribe the nature of documents to accompany such plants and plant materials and articles.
- It authorizes the state governments to make rules for the detention, inspection, disinfection or destruction of any insect or class of insects or any article or class of articles, in respect of which the Central Government has issued notification. It also authorizes the State Governments for regulating the powers and duties of the officers whom it may appoint on its behalf.
- It provides penalty for persons who knowingly contravene the rules and regulations issued under the act.
- It also protects the personnel from any suit or prosecution or other legal proceedings for anything done in good faith as intended to be done under this act.

The quarantine regulations are operative through "The Destructive Insects and Pests Act, 1914 (which has been revised and time from 1930 to 1956 and amended in 1967 and 1992. The Act also empowers the state governments to frame suitable rules and issue notifications for inter-state movement of plant and plant material. Those rules are known as plant quarantine rules. Under the act, Central Government frames rules prescribing the seaports, airports and land frontiers through which plants and specified plant material can enter India, and the manner in which these can be imported. The DIP Act operates under the National Sea Customs Act and the points of entry are located within the jurisdiction of State on the advice of Central Government, the State frames rules for detention, inspection, disinfection and destruction (as against entry) of material, if required, and delegates powers in this regard to concerned authorities with the enforcement of rules.

The Plant Quarantine Service is centrally organized and administered through the Directorate of Plant Protection, Quarantine and Storage established under the Ministry of Agriculture (Department of Agriculture and Co-operation) which is headed by the Plant Protection Adviser to the Government of India and having its headquarters at N.H. IV, Faridabad, Haryana State. When plants are imported there are certain principles which, if followed ensure that as few risks as possible are taken.

- Import from a country where, for the crop in question, pathogens which are mainly to be guarded against are absent.
- Import from a country with an competent plant quarantine service, so that inspection and treatment of planting material before dispatch will be thorough, so reducing the likelihood of contaminated plants being received.
- Take planting material from the safest known source within the chosen country.
- Take an official certificate of freedom from pests and diseases from the exporting country.
- The smaller the amount the less the chance of its carrying infection, and inspection as well as post-entry quarantine.
- Check material watchfully on arrival and treat (dust, spray, fumigate, heat treat) as necessary.
- Import the safest type of planting material, For instance, seeds are usually safer than vegetative material, unrooted cuttings than rooted. axenic cultures of meristem tip tissues (micropropagation).
- If other precautions are not thought to be adequate, the consignment for import should be subject to intermediate or post-entry quarantine. Such quarantine must be carried out at properly equipped station with suitably trained staff.

Seed was not originally included in the DIP Act, but because of the changing circumstances and to meet up the present necessities, the Government of India passed the Plants, Fruits, Seeds (Regulation of Import into Indi(a) Order 1984 which came into effect in June 1985. The conditions for the import of 17 crops are stipulated in this order. The main features of the order are:

1. Seed has been brought under the purview of the DIP Act.
2. No consignment can be imported into the country without valid import permit issued by the Plant Protection Adviser to the Government of India.
3. No consignment can be imported without an official phytosanitary certificate issued by the plant quarantine agency of the exporting country.
4. Post-entry growth of the particular crops at approved locations.

Agencies involved in plant quarantine

The authority to implement the quarantine rules and regulations framed under DIP Act rests basically with the Directorate of Plant Protection, Quarantine & Storage, under the Ministry of Agriculture. This organization handles bulk import and export of seed and planting material for commerical purpose. Under this organization 9 seaports, 10 airports and 7 land frontiers are functioning. These are the recognized ports for entries for import of plant and plant material. The names and places of the ports and stations are as follows.

A. Airports

i. Amritsar - Punjab
ii. Calcutta - West Bengal
iii. Chennai - Tamil Nadu
iv. Hyderabad - Andhra Pradesh
v. Tiruchirappalli - Tamil Nadu
vi. Trivandrum - Kerala
vii. Varanasi - Uttar Pradesh
viii. Mumbai - Maharashtra
ix. New Delhi - New Delhi
x. Patna - Bihar

B. Seaports - Place State / Union territory

i. Bhavnagar - Gujarat
ii. Nagapattinam - Tamil Nadu
iii. Rameswaram - Tamil Nadu
iv. Tuticorin - Tamil Nadu
v. Visakhapatnam - Andhra Pradesh
vi. Calcutta - West Bengal
vii. Chennai - Tamil Nadu
viii. Cochin - Kerala
ix. Mumbai - Maharashtra

C. Land frontiers

i. Bangaon Benapol Border - West Bengal
ii. Gede Road Railway Station - West Bengal
iii. Kalimpong - West Bengal
iv. Sukhia Pokhri - West Bengal
v. Amritsar Railway Station - Punjab
vi. Attari Railway Station - Punjab
viii. Attari-Wagah Border- Punjab

The Government of India has also approved three other national institutions to act as official quarantine agencies, especially for research material.

- **National Bureau of Plant Genetic Resources (NBPGR)**

The NBPGR in New Delhi and its regional station at Hyderabad in the agency involved in processing of germplasm, seed, plant material of agricultural, horticultural, and silvicultural crops of all the institutions of Indian Council of Agricultural Research (ICAR) functioning in the country

- **Forest Research Institute (FRI), Dehra Dun:** for forestry plants
- **Botanical Survey of India (BSI):** for other plants.

Domestic Quarantine

Under the DIP Act, the Directorate of Plant Protection, Quarantine and storage has the accountability to take the essential steps and regulate the inter-state movement of plants and plant material in order to prevent the further spread of destructive pest and diseases that have already entered the country. The solitary object of enforcing domestic quarantine is to prevent the spread of these diseases from infected to non-infected areas. Presently, domestic plant quarantine exists in four diseases, wart (*Synchytrium endobioticum*) of potato from 1959, bunchy top (virus) of banana from 1959, mosaic (virus) of banana from 1961 and apple scab (*Venturia inaequalis*) from 1979. Most of the states in India have plant quarantine laws to avoid entry of plant pests and diseases.

Model Practice Questions

A. Objective Questions

a. Multiple choice Questions

1. Management of plant diseases using legal restriction is called
   - (a) Cultural management
   - (b) Physical management
   - (c) Plant Quarntine
   - (d) Chemical management
2. The term 'Quarantine' is derived from the Latin word *quarantum,* meaning
   - (a) 40
   - (b) 50
   - (c) 60
   - (d) 70
3. Plant quarantine , restrict to protect agriculture and the environment from avoidable damage by hazardous organisms.
   - (a) Entry of plants & plant products
   - (b) Soil, cultures of living organisms
   - (c) Packing materials, commodities, containers and means of conveyance
   - (d) All
4. The first quarantine was imposed in.
   - (a) Venice in 1374
   - (b) Australia in 1374
   - (c) Austria in 1374
   - (d) Purtagal in 1374
5. Strategic and integrated approach encompasses policy frameworks to analyze and manage risks for food safety, animal life, health, and plant life and health including environment
   - (a) Plant Biosecurity
   - (b) Plant Qurantine
   - (c) Agroterrorism
   - (d) Biotererorism
6. Basic elements of plant biosecurity are
   - (a) Introduction of exotic pests/diseases
   - (b) Emergence of virulent strains/races/ biotypes of economically important indigenous pests/diseases
   - (c) Biosafety issues arising from LMOs
   - (d) All

7. Destructive Insects and Pests (DIP) Act was passed in

(a) 1914	(b) 1912
(c) 1910	(d) 1920

8. Introduction of exotic diseases and pests into the country or their spread from one state or union territory to another under

(a) Destructive Insects and Pests (DIP) Act of 1914
(b) Plant Quarantine (Regulations of Import into Indi(a) Order 2003
(c) Livestock Importation Act1898
(d) The Environmental (Protection) Act 1986

9. Which among the following replaces the existing Insecticide act, 1968,

(a) Destructive Insects and Pests (DIP) Act of 1914
(b) Pesticide Management Bill, 2020
(c) Livestock Importation Act1898
(d) The Environmental (Protection) Act 1986

10. Which among the following pests introduced earliest in India

(a) Lantana weed	(b) Coffee rust
(c) Late blight of potato	(d) Wooly apple aphid

11. The benefits derived after taking risk are high enough to justify taking the risk, with safe guards , in the first place.

(a) Low risk pest	(b) High risk pest
(c) Acceptable risk pest	(d) Pest risk analysis

12. Which among the following pests Introduced in 2018 in India

(a) Fall armyworm in maize	(b) White rust of chrysanthemum
(c) Late blight of potato	(d) Wooly aphid of apple

13. Domestic quarantine exist in India for

(a) Potato scab	(b) Potato virus
(c) Potato late blight	(d) Potato wart

14. Once the pathogen has established in an area, steps taken to destroy or remove is known as

(a) Exclusion	(b) Eradication
(c) Protection	(d) Therapy

15. PRA stands for
    (a) Pest restricted area
    (b) Pest risk analysis
    (c) Pest reserved area
    (d) Pesticide risk analysis

Answer

Q. No	Answer	Q. No	Answer
1	(c) Plant Quarntine	7	(a) 1914
2	(a) 40	8	(a) Destructive Insects and Pests (DIP) Act of 1914
3	(d) All	9	(b) Pesticide Management Bill, 2020
4	(a) Venice in 1374	10	(a) Lantana weed
5	(a) Plant Biosecurity	11	(c) Acceptable risk pest
6	(d) All	12	(d) All
13	(d) Potato wart	14	(b) Eradication
15	(b) Pest risk analysis	16	-

b.True/False

1. The basic principles of plant quarantine are to check the entry and spread of potentially dangerous plant pathogens and insects imported along with the germplasm.
2. Low risk pest means that there is little chance that the pathogen or pest will enter.
3. Quarantine regulations are enforced by a country only.
4. Certification is the method of management of pathogen avoiding the contact between the pathogen and the host.
5. Exclusion is the most effective approach to keep pathogens away from the area.
6. The quarantine regulations anticipate that the disease or pathogen is not present in the country.
7. The most used methods for exclusion of the pathogens are regulatory measures.
8. Complete embargo involves absolute prohibition or exclusion of specified plants and plant products from a country infected or infested with highly destructive pests or diseases.
9. Plant quarantine laws were first enacted in India in 1906 in response to concerns about the spread of the Mexican boll weevil.
10. It is not permitted to transport potato tubers from West Bengal to any other state or territory in India because of the possibility of wart spreading.

Answer

Question no	Answer	Question no	Answer
1	True	6	True
2	True	7	True
3	False	8	True
4	True	9	False
5	False	10	True

B.Descriptive Questions

b. Short Answer

1. What is plant quarantine?
2. Why is plant quarantine important?
3. How do plant quarantine regulations vary by country?
4. What are the common methods used in plant quarantine?
5. What is a phytosanitary certificate?

b. Long Answer

1. What is plant quarantine? Describe domestic quarantine measures in India and how they are helpful in crop disease management.
2. What is plant quarantine, and why is it important for global agriculture?
3. What are the main pests and diseases controlled through plant quarantine, and how do they affect crops?
4. Write down the principles and goals of plant quarantine.Give the factors affecting the efficacy of plant quarantines.
5. What are the tow different categories of Plant Quarantine? Give some examples of the plants and plant materials prohibited from entry into India.
6. Explain the process of plant quarantine inspection at ports of entry. What steps are involved in ensuring compliance with quarantine laws?
7. How does plant quarantine contribute to food security and sustainable agriculture?
8. What are the challenges faced by countries in enforcing plant quarantine regulations effectively?
9. Discuss in details about Plant Quarantine organizations in India.
10. Discuss the ethical and environmental considerations of plant quarantine policies. How should governments balance trade with biosecurity concerns?

18

Chemical Management

Anti-pathogen Chemicals

The chemical substances that help to retard the activity of pathogens like fungus, bacteria and nematodes are said to be anti-pathogen chemicals.

Types of anti-pathogen chemicals

Pesticide type	Target pest
Fungicide	Fungi
Insecticide	Insect
Herbicide	Weeds
Acaricide	Mites, Spiders, Ticks
Nematicide	Nematodes
Rodenticide	Rodents

Aim of use of chemicals in plant disease control

The aim and of use of chemicals in plant disease control are

- To create a toxic barrier between the host surface or tissue and the pathogen .
- To eradicate the pathogen present at a particular site on the host, such as seed, foliage, roots etc.

Functions of chemicals in plant disease control

- Reduction in inoculum density or eradication of inoculum from source of growth, multiplication and survival.
- Inactivaion or destruction of the pathogen when it lands on the treated surface, and
- Cure of the diseased plant.

Characters of anti- pathogen chemicals

In general, the anti-infection chemicals or fungicides having following characters are supposed to be ideal.

- High field performance.
- Easy availability of the active constituents.

- Absence of toxicity for the host, man and animals.
- High toxicity for the pathogen at low concentration.
- Retention of toxicity on dilution.
- Stability in storage.
- Slow or no loss of toxicity in storage.
- Good spreading quality on host surface.
- High tenacity on the host surface i.e. it should be retained on the surface.
- Compatibility with pesticides, nematicides, herbicides, vermicides and fertilizers.

Advantages of Employing Chemicals

- **Cost effectiveness**: Pesticides are an economical way of controlling pests. They require low labour input and allow large areas to be treated quickly and effectively. It has been estimated that there is a four-fold return on every rupees a farmer spends on pesticides.
- **Quality, quantity and price of produce**: Using pesticides means there is a plentiful supply and variety of high quality products at reasonable prices. Modern society demands nutritious food free from damage caused by pests and flowers which look untouched. This would be very difficult without pesticides.
- **Prevention of problem**: Pesticides are often used to stop the spread of pests in imports and exports, preventing weeds in gardens and protecting house and furniture from destruction.
- **Protection of pets and humans**: Under the blanket of pesticides is pet flea products, fly and insect spray and other household products which make life bearable.
- **Flexibility**: A suitable pesticide is available for almost all pest problems with variation in type, activity and persistence.
- **Protection of the environment**: Currently, weeds are controlled by herbicides, but without them, land would need to be cultivated, increasing land degradation.

Disadvantages of Employing Chemicals

- **Drift of sprays and vapour**: Pesticides can affect other areas during application and can cause severe problems in different crops, livestock, waterways and the general environment. Wildlife and fish are the most affected.

- **Reduction of beneficial species**: Animals which interact with the targeted pest can also be affected by he chemical application. The reduction in these other organisms can result in changes in the biodiversity of an area and affect natural biological balances.
- **Residues in food**: There is the possibility of pesticides in human food, either by direct application onto the food, or by bio-magnification along the food line. Not all levels are undesirable but unnecessary and dangerous levels must be avoided through good agricultural practice.
- **Contamination of ground water**: Chemicals can reach underground aquifers if there is persistent product use in agricultural areas.
- **Resistance**: Overuse of the same pesticide can encourage resistance in the target pest.
- **Poisoning hazards**: Pesticide operators can risk poisoning through excessive exposure if safe handling procedure are not followed and protective clothing is not worn. Poisoning risks depend on dose, toxicity, duration of exposure and sensitivity.
- **Other possible health effects**: As pesticides used now have been through rigorous testing, most health problems stem from misuse, abuse or overuse.

Classification of Chemicals

There are many chemicals which are available for plant disease control but all are not equally safe, effective and popular. The success of any chemical depends on the selection of suitable chemical and its use at appropriate time and place and its proper application. The chemicals can be broadly classified on the basis of their mode of action against pathogen and type of pathogen.

A. According to mode of action

Depending upon their mode of action the chemicals can be grouped as protectants, eradicants and therapeutants. They are briefly discussed as under.

1. Protectants

Protectants are prophylactic in their nature. These may be applied to seeds, plant surfaces or the soil but cannot penetrate deep into plant tissues. Therefore, they act outside the plant parts as a cover to check the invasion by the pathogen. They include thiram, captan, agallol, zineb, sulphur, ceresan and streptocyclin.

2. Eradicants

Eradicants help to eradicate the dormant or active pathogen from the host completely. They are effective in checking the entry (by covering surfaces) and penetrating in the tissue killing pathogen in the host plant. These chemicals can be used as protectant as well as eradicant. Examples are lime, sulphur, organo mercurials, such as phenyl mercury acetate, methoxy ethyl mercury chloride.

3. Therapeutants

Therapeutants is an agent that inhibits the growth and development of a disease already entered in a plant, when applied appropriately. This therapy can be achieved by physical means, such as solar energy treatment or hot water treatment, but quite often by chemical means and is called chemotherapy. Usually the chemotherapeutants are systemic in their action, i.e. they enter the plants and affect deep seated infection. e.g. plantvax, vitavax, brassicol, dithane M-45, dithane Z- 78, bordeaux mixture, streptocyclin and agromycin.

B. According to type of pathogen

Based on the type of pathogens, the chemicals can be grouped as

(1) Fungicides

(2) Bactericides and

(3) Nematicides

1. Fungicides

The chemicals which kill fungus are called fungicides. Most of the plant diseases are caused by fungus only. Some diseases remain on the surface of the plant while others are deeply seated. These fungicides can again be classified as non systemic and systemic based upon their action in plant.

I. Non- systemic or Contact fungicides

Non-systemic or contact fungicides are the chemicals which do not enter inside the plant tissue, but kill the pathogen by surface contact. Some of the important categories of chemicals used for disease control are given here.

A. Sulphur fungicides

Sulphur fungicides are the oldest method of disease control. Inorganic sulphur is used in the form of elemental sulphur or as lime sulphur mixture. Elemental sulphur can be in dust form or. as wettable powder, the latter is used more commonly. However, the most popular fungicides in sulphur groups are the organic compounds known as dithio-carbamates. .Some of the important chemicals under dithiocarbamates are thiram, ferbam, ziram, nabam, zineb and maneb.

1. Thiram

The trade name for thiram is arasan, tundas, terson, tulisan, etc. It is a leading chemical for seed treatment . It is also used in the control of foliage disease Pythium, Rhizoctonia, Fusarium and Protomyces.

2. Zineb

Zineb is also known as dithane Z- 78, parzate or lonacol. It is effective as foliar spray against late blight of potatoes and tomatoes, blast of rice, ripe rot of chillies and downey mildew of maize.

3. Maneb

Maneb is called as dithane M-22, manzate or dithane M-45. It is effective against bean anthracnose caused by Colletorrichum spp. downy mildew and anthracnose of cucurbits, fruit rot of chillies, citrus greasy spot maize leaf blight, and blights caused by Alternaria, Phytophthora and Cercospora on crops.

B. Copper fungicides

Bordeaux and Burgundy mixtures are the dispersible forms of cuprous oxide and basic carbonates are among the important copper fungicides.

1. Bordeaux mixture

Bordeaux mixture (5: 5 : 50) is prepared as

Ingredient	Quantity
Copper sulphate (Blue stone)	5lb (2.26 kg)
Stone or hydrated lime	5 lb (2.26 kg)
Water	50 gallons

It is specific against downy mildew, late blight of potato, coffee rust, various leaf spots diseases, blights, anthracnoses etc.

2. Burgundy mixture

Burgundy mixture is also known as "Soda bordeaux" It is prepared as.

Ingredient	Quantity
Copper sulphate (Blue stone)	10 lb (4.5 kg)
Stone or hydrated lime	12.21b (5.6 kg)
Water	50 gallons.

3. Chestnut compound

Chestnut compound contains two parts of copper sulphate and 11 parts of ammonium carbonate. The two substances are well powdered and thoroughly mixed and the dry mixture stored in an airtight receptacle for 24 hours before being used. It is used against damping -off disease.

4. Chaubattia paste

Chaubattia paste is prepared by mixing copper carbonate -800 g, red lead -800 g and raw linseed oil or lanolin -1littre. This paste was developed as a wound dressing fungicide to be applied to pruned parts of pears, apples and peaches for the control of disease, such as stem black, stem-brown, pink disease, stem canker and collar rot of apples, peaches, apricots and plums.

C. Mereury fungicides

Many mercury compounds are highly effective as fungicides and bactericides. Mercuric chloride (Hg CI_2) and mercurous chloride (Hg_2C1_2) are used as 1 : 1000 dilutions for soaking the seeds, rhizomes and corms of vegetables and flowers to mainly control certain bacterial and fungal diseases. It is used against club root disease of Brassica seedlings.

D. Quinone fungicides

Some common quinone fungicides are mentioned here.

1. Chloranil

Chloranil is mainly used in seed treatment. It is sold as spergon and is used in seed and bulb treatment of legume flowers and vegetables. It is also used as soil drench.

2. Dichlone

Dichlone is used as seed treatment as well as foliar spray also. It is 4-8 times more effective than chloranil in the protection of legume and cotton seed.

E. Benzene fungicides

Benzene is used as a dormant spray for the control of many diseases of fruit trees and ornamental plants and for the treatment of wounds in trees.

1. Dinocap (Karathane)

Dinocap is an excellent substitute for sulphur for the control of powdery mildew and is highly specific against them. It is also effective against mites.

2. Chloronil

Chloronil is active against *Rhizoctonia solani; Sclerotium rolfsii* and *Phytophthora cinnamoni*. This fungicide has been used for the most part as a seed or in-furrow treatment of cotton.

3. Penta chloronitrobenzene (PCNB)

Penta chloronitrobenzene is sold as quintozene, PCNB, terrachlor, brassicol etc. They control many soil-borne diseases. PCNB acts by preventing sporulation. Diseases caused by Rhizoctonia, Sclerotium etc. are controlled by PCNB.

F. Hetero-cyclic nitrogen compound

Hetero-cyclic nitrogen compound are used as foliage protectants and eradicants of fruits and vegetables. Glyodin and captan are the two important fungicides of this group.

1. Captan

Captan is sold under different names like capton orthocide dust etc. It is effective for seed treatment for seedling diseases of vegetables, cotton etc, smuts, and bunt wheat. It is also used as spray fungicide against, downy mildew and powdery mildew of grapevines, apple scab, brown rot of stone fruits and mango anthracnose.

2. Difoltan

Difoltan has properties similar to captan. It is a good fungicide for the control of early and late blight of potatoes and tomatoes.

3. Folpet

It is sold under the trade names of phaltan, orthophaltan etc. Wettable powder and dust are applied for foliage diseases of fruits and ornamentals. Folpet is eftective against *Sphaerotheca pannosa.*

G. Organo-phophorus fungicides

1. Ediphenphos

It is the common name to the fungicide sold under the trade name Hinosan. It is an effective against blast of rice.

H. Organo- tin compounds

1. Brestan

Brestan is effective against *Cercospora, Alternaria*, *Spetoria* and many other fungi.

2. Du-Ter

Du-Ter is used effectively against diseases caused by *Cercospora, Helminthosporium, Alternaria*, *Pythium, Phytophthora* and *Rhizoctonia.*

I. Soil fumigants

The most promising method of controlling nematodes in the field has been through the use of chemicals called nematicides. Some of these, including chloropicrin, methyl bromide, vapam and vorlex, give off gases after being applied ; to the soil. Some of the soil fumigants are mentioned here.

1. Formalin

Formalin is used to control damping-off and seedling blights. A solution of 37-40% in water is used.

2. Chloropicrin

Chloropicrin is useful both as a fungicide and a larvicide. It is injected into the soil at a depth of 3-6" in holes 9-12" apart. The soil is then covered with impervious cloth or sheet for 48 hours.

3. Vapam

Vapam is a colourless liquid which decomposes rapidly in moist soil to release a fumigating gas. It has been used as nematicide and also as selective weedicide. It is also quite effective in the control of wilt of cotton, damping-off of papaya and root rot of beet.

4. DD Mixture (Dichloropropene and Dichloropropane)

DD Mixture is extensively used as nematode control. Also used as control of soil borne diseases in pineapple.

II. Systemic fungicides

Sysyemics fungicides are the fungicitoxic compounds which when applied on different parts of the plant are absorbed by the plant tissues and then translocated upwards, downwards and both ways and act on the pathogen either directly or through its metabolite products and control plant diseases away from the point of application .

An ideal systemic fungicide should have the following characteristics.

1. The substance may either be toxic to the pathogen concerned or be converted in the host plant to such a fungitoxicant.
2. Alternatively, the substance may alter the metabolism of the host so that biochemical or physical resistance to pathogen may be induced or enhanced.
3. It must not adversely affect the host plant to such an extent that the quantity or quality of the crop is reduced.
4. Systemic fungicides are highly selective i.e. toxic to the pathogen but not to the host .
5. In systemicity the substance must be absorbed sufficiently the translocated from the point of application to the site of the pathogen and should have a considerable degree of stability within the host plant.

6. Most systemic fungicides are translocated in the apoplast , though some mainly compound related to the benzimidazoles, appear to move in the symplast also.
7. Systemic fungicides are advantageous over non systemic fungicides because of more coverage, systemic and mobile nature.so that concealed pathogens are also targeted, more specific in mode of action and thus less quantity is required against fast growing fungi.
8. However, there are some disadvantages also like narrow spectrum of activity, development of resistance of pathogen, higher cost and residual toxicity if it is not metabolized in the system.
9. If it is applied to an edible portion of the plant the mammalian toxicity must be low enough to avoid residue problems at the consumer stage.

On the basis of chemical structure, systemic fungicides can be classified as follows.

1. Oxathins and related compounds

These were the first systemic fungicides to be discovered in 1966. They selectively concentrate in cells of fungi and inhibit succinic hydrogenase (enzyme involved in mitochondrial respiration). Oxathins are systemic fungicides which are effective only against Basidiomycetous fungi, such as Rusts, Smuts, Rhizoctonia etc. Two types of oxathins are there.

a. Vita vax or Carboxin

Vitavax or carboxin has become the most popular fungicide for seed treatment to control loose smut in wheat and barley. It gives satisfactory control of bunt and flag smut also.

b. Plant vax or Oxycarboxin

Plant vax or Oxycarboxin is toxic to *Helminthosporium sativum*, *Curvularia, Aspergillus, Eladosporium, Botrytis, Monilinia* etc.

2. Benzimidazoles

Benzimidazole fungicides were introduced for disease control in the 1960s and 197 as foliar fungicides, seed treatments and for use in post harvest applications. They possessed unique properties not seen before in the protectants. These includes low use rates, broad spectrum and systemicity with post infection action that allowed for extended spray interval. All these qualities made them very popular with growers. These fungicide show broad spectrum activity against fungi but are not effective against lower fungi and bacteria.

a. Benomyl

This is also marketed as benlate. It is effective against *Cercospora* leaf spot of sugarbeet, rice blast, apple scab, powdery mildew of curubits, cereals and legumes. Dipping of fruits and roots has controlled banana fruit rots, root rot of sweet potato, corn rot of gladiolus etc

b. Carbendazim

Carbendazim is effective against a wide range of fungal pathogens of field crops, fruits, ornamentals and vegetables as spray, seedling dip, seed treatment, soil drench and as post harvest treatment.It is very effective against wilt diseases,, turmeric leaf spot and rust diseases.

c. Thiabendazole (TBZ)

It is sold as Thiabendazole, Mertect, Tecto, Storite. Thiabendazole is a broad spectrum systemic fungicide effective against species of *Botrytis, Ceratocystis, Coleetotrichum, Fusarium, Cercospora, Rhizoctonia, Sclerotinia, Septoria* and *Verticillium.* It is also used to control post harvest storage diseases of fruits and vegetables.

3. Acylalanines

These are was introduced in 1977, brought a completely new level of control to oomycetes through their systemic properties by offering protection to the plants as seed treatments, soil or foliar applications. These include metalaxyl, furalaxyl or banalaxyl. These fungicides are highly effective against downy mildews, *Pythium* and *Phytophthora* diseases including late blight.

4. Thiophanates

These compounds are the derivatives of thioallophanic acid representing a new group of systemic fungicides. The aromatic nucleus of these fungicides is converted into benzimidazole ring for their activity. Hence, thiophanates are often classified under benzimidazole group.Two compounds are developed under this group are Thiophanate and Thiophanate –methyl .The former has a broad range of action and is effective against *Venturia* spp. on apple and pear, powdery mildews, *Botrytis* and *Sclerotinia* spp.Thiophanate methyl is also recommended for use in the management of apple scab, powdery mildews and some leaf spots.

5. Morpholines

Morpholine fungicides are best known for their excellent control of cereal diseases, powdery mildew on vegetable and grapes, and sigatoka of banana. Tridemorph and Dodemorph are the common morpholine fungicides sold as Calixin ,Bradew and Beacon etc. Among the recently developed systemic fungicides, Tridemorph has excellent prophylactic and curative action against powdery mildew of cereals, sigatoka disease of banana and other ascomycetous pathogens. Dodemorph is widely used in the management of powdery mildew of roses.

6. Sterol biosynthesis inhibitor(SBIs) fungicides

SBIs have proved most successful fungicides for about three decades since their release in 1970's. Their mode of action is inhibition of sterol (ergosterol) biosynthesis, an important component of cell membranes of Asco- and Basidiomycotina.Sterol biosynthesis inhibitor fungicides include Pyrimidines, Piperidines, Imidazole and Piperazine. Among all SBIs, triazoles are the most commonly used. Triazoles are one of the most effective fungicides such as triadimefon (Bayleton,) and triadimenol (Baytan), both of which are effective against powdery mildews. Others in this group are hexaconazole (Contaf 5EC, Anvil 5 EC), triazbutyl (Indar or RH 124) , propiconazole (Tilt 25 EC) and terbuconazole (Folicur 25 EC) etc. In addition to powdery mildew , hexaconazole is effective against rusts, propiconazole against rust and leaf spots, terbuconazole as seed treatment fungicide against smuts, penconazole and difenoconazole and cyperocoanazole against leaf spots and rusts and porbenazole is specific against rice blast.

7. Strobilurins fungicides

Strobilurins are a group of chemical compounds used in agriculture as fungicides. They were extracted from the fungus *Strobilurus tenacellus* and hence the name strobilurin. These fungicides have become very important in the control of wide range of plant diseases caused by all major groups of fungi, Asco, Basidio, and the Oomycota. They have a suppressive effect on other fungi, reducing competition for nutrients; they inhibit electron transfer in mitochondria, disrupting energy metabolism and preventing growth of the target fungi. They are part of the larger group of QoI inhibitors, which act to inhibit the respiratory chain at the level of Complex III. Some common Strobilurins are azoxystrobin, kresoxim-methyl, picoxystrobin, fluoxastrobin, oryzastrobin, dimoxystrobin, pyraclostrobin and trifloxystrobin. Strobilurins represented a major development in fungus-based fungicides. Strobilurins are miracle fungicides ever developed.

Pesticide Formulations

Defnition

Pesticide formulation is the process by which the pesticide is put into a form which can be easily produced, stored, transported and applied by practical methods in order to achieve a safe, convenient economic and effective method of pest control.

When a pesticide active ingredient (a.i) is manufactured, it is not in a usable form as it may not mix well with water or may be unstable. Therefore, it is mixed with other compounds to improve its effectiveness, safety, handling and storage. These other compounds can include solvents, mineral clays, stickers, wetting agents, or other adjuvant. The mixture of active and inert (inactive) ingredients is called a pesticide formulation. Some formulations are premixed while others must be mixed before use. A single a.i. is often made into several formulations.

Objectives of Pesticide Formulations

The objective of formulating pesticide active ingredients for crop protection is:

- To uniformly spread a small amount of the active ingredient over a large area.
- To ensure safety in handling and application.
- To optimize pesticide doses for better efficacy.

How to Choose a Formulation?

Selection of the most appropriate formulation for a given application includes an analysis of the following factors:

Application safety: Different formulations create varied degrees of hazards for the applicator. Some products are easily inhaled, while others may readily penetrate skin, or cause injury when splashed in the eyes.

Pest biology: The growth habits and survival strategies of pests are also key factors in determining which type of formulation provides optimum contact between the active ingredients and the pest.

Environmental concern: Special precautions need to be taken with formulations that are prone to drift in the air or move off target into water. Wildlife may also be affected in varying degrees by different formulations.

Available application equipment: Some pesticide formulations require specialized application equipment. This includes safety equipment and , in special cases, containment structures.

Surface to be protected: Applicators must be aware that certain formulations can stain fabrics, discolor linoleum, dissolve plastic, or burn foliage. These surfaces require protection.

Cost: Product prices may vary substantially, based on the ingredients used and the complexity of delivering active ingredients in specific formulations.

Conventional Pesticide Formulations

Solid formulations: These are divided into t types: ready to use, and concentrates which must be mixed with water in order to be applied as spray able suspensions. Of the six solid formulations dust, granules, and pellets are ready to use, while other three wettable powders, dry flowable powders, and soluble powders are intended to be mixed with water before applying in the field.

Dusts: These are manufactured by the sorption of an active ingredient onto a finely ground, solid inert such as clay, chalk or talc. Usually the concentration of active ingredients in these formulations is less than 10%.

A granule is defiend by size. Granule sized products should pass through a 4 mesh sieve and be retained on an 80 mesh sieve.

Granules: The manufacture of granular formulations is similar to that of dusts except that the active ingredient is sorbed onto a larger particle. The inert solid may be clay, sand or ground plant materials. Granules are applied in the dry state and are usually intended for soil applications where they have the advantage of weight to carry them through foliage to the ground below.

Pellets: The active ingredient is combined with inert materials to form slurry (a thick liquid mixture) and the slurry is then extruded under pressure through a die and cut at desired lengths to produce particles that are relatively uniform in size and shape. These pellets are typically used in spot applications.

Wettable powders: These powders are finely divided solids made of mineral clays to which an active ingredient is mixed and sorbed. These formulations are diluted with water and applied as a liquid spray. Under dilution, a suspension is formed in the spray tank. Apart from the active ingredient, wettable powders contain wetting and dispersing agents as an inert part of the formulation.

Dry flowable or water dispersible granules: They are diluted with water and applied as a spray suspension exactly in the same manner as wettable powders and dry flowables are expected to form a stable suspension with high susceptibility and they are also considered more environment and user friendly in comparison with wettable powders.

Soluble powders: Soluble powders provide most of the same benefits as wettable powders, without they need for agitation once they are dissolved in the spray tank.

Liquid formulations: There are four types of liquid formulations available in the market. Prior to application these are diluted with water, but in some instances labels may permit the use of crop, oil, diesel fuel, kerosene, or some other light fuel oil as carrier. The four different types are:

Emulsifiable Concentrates: These are non aqueous solutions of pesticide along with emulsifiers, which, on dilution with water, produce a stable emulsion. Emulsifiable concentrates are mixed with water and applied as a spray. The emulsifing agents are long chain chemicals that oreint themselves around the droplets of oil and bind the oil water surfaces together to prevent the oil and water from separating. Emulsifiable concentrates allow oil soluble active ingredients to be sprayed in the field using water as a carrier.

Liquid Flowables: The manufacture of liquid flowable mirrors that of wattable powders with the additional step of mixing the powder, dispersing agents, wetting agents, etc., with water followed by wet grinding for making a stable suspension before packaging.

Microencapsulators: Microencapsulates consist of a solid and liquid inert, containing an active ingredient surrounded by a plastic, starch or polymers coating. The resulting capsules can be aggregated to form dispersible granules, or they may be suspended in water to form a capsulated suspension. Encapsulation enhances applicator safety along with minimization of residues, while at the same time providing timed release of the active ingredient. Liquid forms of microencapsulates are further diluted with water and applied as sprays. They form suspensions in the spray tank and have several properties similar to those of the liquid flowable.

Solutions: (Water soluble concentrates) These consists of water soluble active and inert ingredients to be used for further dilutions prior to field applications. They form a true solution in the spray tank and require no agitation after they are thoroughly dissolved. Solutions are not abrasive to equipment and donot plug strainers and screens. They include products containing paraquat, glyphosate and 2,4-D.

Aerosols and Fumigants: Aerosols really refers to a delivery system that moves the active ingredient to the target site in the form of a mist of very small particles. The particles can be released under pressure or produced by fog or smoke generators. Fumigants deliver the active ingredient to the target site in the form of a gas. Some fumigants are solids that sublime (turn into gas) in the presence of atmospheric moisture. Others are liquid under pressure that vaporizes when the pressure is released.

Disadvantages of Conventional Formulations	**Advantages of New Generation Formulations**
Bulky, dusty and inconvenient	Improved residual activity
Hazardous during manufacturing, packing and application	Longer application intervals
Highly flammable due to use of organic solvents	Reduction in application dosage

Disadvantages of Conventional Formulations	Advantages of New Generation Formulations
Can cause phytotoxicity	Reduction in spray drift
More impact on non target organism	Less impact on non target organisms
Poor rain fastness	Better rain fastness
Corrosive to metal and plastic	Less phytotoxicity
Expensive to pack and transport	Constant and delayed biological effect
Dermal hazards	Reduced environmental pollution
Extreme inhalation danger	Reduced volatilization and leaching
	Safe storage due to reduced flammability

Fungicide Resistance

Fungicides have been used for over 200 years to protect plants against fungal diseases. At present about 150 chemicals belonging to different classes are used as fungicides in world agriculture. Most of the recommended treatments generally provide 90% or greater control of the target disease, and give the farmer a benefit: cost ratio of at least 3:1. However, under certain circumstances, a fungicide might fail to control disease development. Poor disease control with fungicides can result from numerous causes, including inherently low fungicide effectiveness, inappropriate timing of application, inadequate dose, faulty method of application, longer interval between applications, expired product or exceedingly heavy disease pressure. Development of resistance to fungicides can also be the reason of poor disease control. *Resistance refers to a situation where a given fungicide once controlled a particular fungal population but, after one or more applications that fungicide no longer controls that population. Resistance to fungicides has become a challenging problem in the management of crop diseases and has threatened the performance of some highly potent commercial fungicides*. Worldwide, resistance in pathogen populations to more than 100 different active ingredient has been reported. The first case of resistance to benzimidazoles occurred in powdery mildew in greenhouses in 1969 in New York, one year after introduction . Resistance to benzimidazioles has been reported to occur in about 126 fungal species including member of the basidiomycetes, ascomycetes and deuteromycetes. Prior to the introduction of benzimidazoles, (benomyl), farmers normally applied protectant fungicides *viz* dithiocarbamates without experiencing resistance problems and these are still used extensively and efficiently against several diseases. Superior disease control was frequently achieved with benomyl compared to the protective dithiocarbamates owing to its systemic activity. However within the few years wherever these fungicide was used intensively, sudden failures in control of disease were experienced with apple scab, powdery mildews, botrytis grey mould and peanut leaf spot.

Majority of the fungicides developed and registered since the introduction of benzimidazoles have site specific mode of actions and carry risk of resistance. Therefore, strategies to manage the resistance risk need to be developed and implemented to avoid unexpected control failures and sustain the usefulness of new products.

Instances of resistance development to compounds of major classes of fungicides used in plant disease control.

Fungicide group/compound	Main Pathogens affected	References
Benomyl	*Botrytis cinerea*	Grape
Carbendazim	*Venturia inaequalis*	Apple
Metalaxyl	*Pseudoperonospora cubensis*	Cucurbits
	Plasmopara viticola	Grapes
	Phytophthora infestans	Potato
	Bremia lactucae	Lettuce
	Botrytis cinerea	Strawberry
	Corynespora cassiicola	Cucumber
	Botrytis cinerea	Grapes
	Alternaria alternata	Oil seeds
	Venturia inaequalis	Apple
	Sclerospora fuliginea	Cucurbit and Barley
	Mycosphaerella graminicola.	Cereal
Edifenphos	*Magnoporthe grisea*	Rice
Ethirimol	*Erysiphe graminis*	Barley
	Alternaria solani	Potato
	Colletotrichum graminicola	Barley
	Cercospora sojina	Soybean

Types of Fungicide Resistance

There are two types of fungicide resistance:

Qualitative resistance (Discreate resistance): Develops suddenly against fungicides that have a single site of action. A mutation in the gene of the target site alters the site of action of the fungicide that makes the fungicide totally ineffective the pathogen. The resistance is stable and persists even after the fungicide is withdrawn. This type of resistance is seen with the use of benzimidazoles and QoI (Strobilurin) fungicides. A point mutation (single nucleotide change) in the gene encoding cytochrome b makes Mycospharella musicola resistant to QoI fungicides, which causes the Sigatoka disease in bananas. The aminoacid glycine is replaced by aniline in the target protein (cytochrome b). The fungicide fails to bind to the protein and becomes ineffective.

Quantitative resistance (Continuous resistance): Develops gradually and is the result of accumulation of mutations in several genes(polygenic), each having a small additive effects.There is a continuous variation in sensitivity within the resistant population. The resistance is not present and the pathogens become sensitive again if the fungicide application is stopped. The DMI (demethylation inhibitor) fungicides induce quantitative resistance.

Preexisting resistance: Besides qualitative and quantitative resistance, caused by monogenic and polygenic mutations respectively, the resistance could be by inbuilt in mechanisms. The apple scab fungus, *Venturia inaequalis* develops resistance against DMI fungicides by upregulation of the target genes, resulting in hyperproduciton of the target proteins and making the fungicide less effective. Efflux of the fungicide out of the cell is reported in *Mycospharella.*

Resistance risk among fungicides

The risk of resistance development depends greatly upon the chemical class to which a fungicvide belongs and the mode of action of member fungicides. Over the past thirty years severe and wide spread problems of acquired resistance have affected the practical performance of most of the major groups of fungicides. Certain traditional major classes of fungicides such as those based on copper (cuprous oxide, copper oxychloride, bordeaux mixture), phthalimides (e.g captan, captafol and folpet) and dithiocarbamates (e.g. mancozeb, maneb, zineb and thiram) have never been known to encounter practical resistance even after many years of use. These fungicides have a multisite mode of action, so that a number of simultaneous mutations would be needed in order to develop resistance. By contrast, all the compounds in some other classes, such as benzimidazoles e.g. benomyl, carbendazim, thiabendazole, pheylamides (e.g. metalxyl and oxadixyl), dicarboximides (e.g. iprodione, peocymidoneand, vinclozolin) and the recently introduced strobilurins (e.g. azoxystrobin and kresoxim methyl) have met with serious resistance problems that arose in most of their target pathogens, within 2-10 years of their commercial introduction. Resistance to triazoles (e.g. triadimefon or flusilazole) has developed more gradually in stepwise process. Estimates of resistance risk in different chemical classes of fungicides are shown in Table-2

Fungicides grouped by mode of action and relative risk for developing resistance problems.

Group name	Mode of action	Common Name	Mobility[1]	Uses[2]	Risk[3]
Phenylamide	Nucleic acid synthesis	Metalaxyl	S	ST, F, S	H
		Metalaxyl-M	S	ST, F, S	H
Benzimidazole	Mitosis and Cell divison	Thiophanate-methyl	S	ST, PH	H
		Thiabendazole	S	ST, F, S	H
Carboxamide	Respiration	Carboxin	S	ST	L
Strobilurin	Respiration	Azoxystrobin	S	F, S, ST	H
Quinone inside Inhibitor	Respiration	Cyazofamid	S	F	M
Dicarboximide	Lipids and membranes	Iprodione	P	F, S	M-H
		Vinclozolin	P	F, S	M-H
	Aromatic hydrocarbons	Chloroneb	P	ST	L
Demethylation Inhibitor (DMI)	Sterol synthesis	Cyproconazole	S	F	
		Difenconazole	S	ST, F	L-M
		Propiconazole	S	F, S	M
		Prothioconazole	S	F,S	M
		Tebuconazole	S	F, S, ST	M
		Triadimefon	S	F, S	M
		Triadimenol	S	ST	L
Cyanoacetamide-oxime	Unknown	Cymoxanil	S	F	M
Phosphonate	Unknown	Fosetyl-AL	S	F	L
Inorganic	Multi-site	Copper salts, Sulphur	P	F	L
Dithiocarbamate	Multi-site	Ferbam, Ziram	P	F	L
		Mancozeb ,Maneb, Thiram	P	F, ST	L
Phthalimide	Multi-site	Captan	P	F, ST	L
Chloronitrile	Multi-site	Chlorothalonil	P	F, S	L
Guanadin	Multi-site	Dodine	P	F	M

Source: http://osufacts.okstate.edu

1. P= Protectant, S = Systemic or penetrant.
2. S = Soilborne diseases, F = Foliar diseases, ST = Seed treatment, PH = Post-harvest treatment.
3. H-High Resistance, M-Moderate resistance, L-Low resistance

Mechanisms of Fungicide Resistance

There are several ways that populations of fungi can become resistant to fungicides, these include:

1. **Altered target site**: A fungicide has a specific target site where it acts to disrupt a particular biochemical process or function. If this target site is somewhat altered, the fungicide no longer binds to the site of action and is unable to exert its toxic effect. This is the most common mechanism that fungi use to become resistant
2. **Detoxification of metabolism**: Metabolism within the fungal cell is one mechanism a disease pathogen uses to detoxify a foreign compound such as a fungicide. A fungus with the ability to quickly degrade a fungicide can potentially inactivate it before it can reach its site of action.
3. **Removal:** A fungal cell may rapidly export the fungicide before it can reach the target site of action.
4. **Reduced uptake of fungicide**: The resistant pathogen simply absorbs the fungicide much more slowly than the susceptible.

Resistance Management

There are several ways to retard the development of resistance.These include:

1. **Tank mix with a fungicide with a different mode of action**. Mancozeb or chlorothalonil can be tank mixed effectively with benzimidazole or phenylamide fungicides.
2. **Apply a limited number of applications in a block at a critical period in the pathogen disease cycle**. A different mode of action should be used at other less critical times in the disease cycle, so as to minimize the exposure of the "at risk" fungicide. This has been recommended with some of the strobilurins.
3. **Alternate applications between or among two or more classes of fungicides with different modes of action**. This is a good strategy for resistance management of triphenyltin hydroxide, the sterol inhibitors, the dicarboximides and the strobilurins. Although the sterol inhibitors and the phenylamides have some post-infection activity, they are best used in a preventive manner, which reduces the likelihood that resistance will develop.
4. **Limit the number of applications of an "at risk" fungicide per year**. This has been done with the phenylamide fungicides, the sterol inhibitors, and the strobilurins. Use of these fungicides may be restricted to the most critical parts of the season.

5. **Avoid reduced rates of fungicides.** These reduced rates may facilitate the development of resistance in fungi.
6. Do not use phenylamides as soil treatments against airborne pathogens.

Methods of application of Fungicides

Proper selection of a fungicide and its application at the correct dose and the proper time are highly essential for the management of plant diseases. The basic requirement of an application method is that it delivers the fungicide to the site where the active compound will prevent the fungus damaging the plant. The fungicidal application varies according to the nature of the host part diseased and nature of survival and spread of the pathogen. The method which are commonly adopted in the application of the fungicides are discussed

1. Foliar or vegetative application

Applying chemicals on the stem, leaves, flowers and fruits is called foliar or vegetative application. Foliar application is carried out in the form of spray, dust or paste.

a. Spraying

This is the most commonly followed method. Spraying of fungicides is done on leaves, stems and fruits. Formulations available in wettable powder, solution or emulsified form are used for spraying. The amount of spray solution required for a hectare will depend on the nature of crops to be treated. For trees and shrubs more amount of spray solution is required than in the case of ground crops. Depending on the volume of fluid used for coverage, the sprays are categorized into high volume, medium volume, low volume, very high volume and ultra low volume. The different equipments used for spray application are: Foot-operated sprayer, rocking sprayer, knapsack sprayer, motorised knapsack sprayer (Power sprayer), tractor mounted sprayer, mist blower and aircraft or helicopter (aerial spray).Generally, these chemicals are dissolved in water and sprayed using a pressure pump. Spraying of chemicals is more prevalent for controlling fungal diseases of foliage.

b. Dusting

Dusts are applied to leaves, stems and fruits of plants. It is used during wet weather which favours sticking of the chemical on the plant surface. Dry powders are used for covering host surface. The equipments employed for the dusting operation are: Bellow duster, rotary duster, motorised knapsack duster and aircraft (aerial application).

c. Pasting and painting

Chemicals are occasionally mixed with water, alcohol, or other carriers and applied as a paint on injured surface or parts of the plant. When trees are pruned, application of paste or paint is necessary. For example, Bordeaux mixture can be made into a paint or slurry with linseed oil or water and can be applied to the cut portions of the trees.

2. Soil treatment

The aim of soil treatment with chemical is to eradicate or reduce plant pathogen population which is harboured in the soil. But the complete eradication of pathogen from soil is not feasible because of degradation of chemicals by physical, chemical and biological means. The soil treatment can be done by drenching of soil with solution or emulsion, and broadcasting of dusted granules.

a. Drenching

Chemicals mainly fungicides are mixed with water at the same concentration as for foliar spraying i.e. 0.01 to 0.03 per cent. The solution is applied to the soil surface either before or after planting. The sprinkled material should reach the depth of at least 10-15 cm. This method is followed for controlling damping off, root rots, seedling blight or infection at the ground level.

b. Broadcasting of dusted granules

Sometimes non-volatile fungicides mixed with soil or fertilizer are scattered with hands as uniformly as possible over the field. They are mixed with the soil up to plough sole in depth. I.e. up to 6 inches by light ploughing or harrowing. This method is too expensive, since it requires a large quantity of chemicals.

c. Furrow application

The chemicals are applied in the furrows in the form of dusts and granules. This method is possible only in crop plants which are in furrows, such as, potato and sugarcane.

d. Fumigation

Application of certain chemicals to the soils can control fungi and nematodes. Such chemicals produce a gas that distributes itself through soil and are called volatile chemicals. By the release of gas, they kill the larvae of nematodes and other pathogens present in the soil. Applications of these highly toxic volatile substances is recommended some weeks before actual planting of crops. Methyle bromide, ethylene dibromide (EDB) and ED/CT mixture are examples of fumigants. The depth of application is maintained at 15-20cm. A thin polythene sheet is required to confine the gas to the soil. This method is usually restricted to small areas.

d. Chemigation

In this method, the fungicides are directly mixed in the irrigation water. It is normally adopted using sprinkler or drip irrigation system.

3. Seed treatment

The concept of seed treatment is the use and application of biological and chemical agents that control or contain primary soil and seed borne infestation of insect pests and diseases which otherwise causes considerable economic loss to crop production or productivity. Seed treatment is definitely a more safe and judicious use of agrochemicals. Treatment of seed results in good establishment of healthy plants leading to better yield. There are various types of seed treatment and broadly they may be divided into three categories (a) Mechanical, (b) Chemical and (c) Physical.

A. Mechanical method

Some pathogen when attack the seeds, there may be alteration in size, shape and weight of seeds by which it is possible to detect the infected seeds and separate them from the healthy ones. In the case of ergot diseases of bajra, rye, sorghum, the fungal sclerotia are usually larger in size and lighter than healthy grains. So by sieving or flotation, the infected grains may be easily separated. Such mechanical separation eleminates the infected grains may be easily separated. Such mechanical separation eliminates the infected materials to a larger extent. Eg. Removal of ergot in sorghum seeds. Dissolve 2kg of common salt in 10 litres of water (20% solution). Drop the seeds into the salt solution and stir well. Remove the ergot affected seeds and sclerotia which float on the surface. Wash the seeds in fresh water 2 or 3 times to remove the salts on the seeds. Dry the seeds in shade and use for sowing. This method is also highly useful to separate infected grains in the case of „tundu‟ disease of wheat.

B. Chemical methods

Using fungicides on seed is one of the most efficient and economical methods of chemical disease control. On the basis of their tenacity and action, the seed dressing chemicals may be grouped as (i) Seed disinfectant, are those which destroy the pathogen that has already infected the seed and established itself in the tissues. (ii) Seed disinfestants, which kill or inactivate the fungus or bacterium present on the seed but do not remain active for long after the seed has been planted and (iii) Seed protectants, which disinfect the seed surface and stick to the seed surface for sometime after the seed has been sown, thus giving temporary protection to the young seedlings against soil borne fungi. Now, the systemic fungicides are impregnated into the seeds to eliminate the deep seated infection in the seeds. The seed dressing chemicals may be applied by (i) Dry treatment (ii) Wet treatment and (iii) Slurry.

(i) Dry Seed Treatment

In this method, the fungicide adheres in a fine from on the surface of the seeds. A calculated quantity of fungicide is applied and mixed with seed using machinery specially designed for the purpose. The fungicides may be treated with the seeds of small lots using simple Seed treating drum or of large seed lots at seed processing plants using Grain treating machines. Normally in field level, dry seed treatment is carried out in dry rotary seed treating drums which ensure proper coating of the chemical on the surface of seeds. Eg. Dry seed treatment in paddy. Mix a required amount of fungicide with required quantity of seeds in a seed treating drum or polythene lined gunny bags, so as to provide uniform coating of the fungicide over the seeds. Treat the seeds atleast 24 hours prior to soaking for sprouting. Any one of the following chemical may be used for treatment at the rate of 2g/kg : Thiram or Captan or Carboxin or Tricyclazole. In addition, the dry dressing method is also used in pulses, cotton and oil seeds with the antagonistic fungus like *Trichoderma vitide* by mixing the formulation at the rate of 4g/kg of the seed.

(ii) Wet seed treatment

This method involves preparing fungicide suspension in water, often at field rates and then dipping the seeds or seedlings or propagative materials for a specified time. The seeds cannot be stored and the treatment has to be done before sowing. This treatment is usually applied for treating vegetatively propagative materials like cuttings, corms, tubers, setts, rhizomes, bulbs etc., which are not amenable to dry or slurry treatment.

a. Seed soaking

Seed soaking is essential for certain crops. Seeds treated by these methods have to be properly dried after treatment. The fungicide adheres as a thin film over the seed surface which gives protection against invasion by soil-borne pathogens. Eg. Seed dip treatment in Wheat. Prepare 0.2% of carboxin solution (2g/litre of water) and soak the seeds for 6 hours. Drain the solution and dry the seeds properly before sowing. This effectively eliminates the loose smut pathogen, *Ustilago tritici.* Eg. Seed dip treatment in paddy. Prepare the fungicidal solution by mixing any of the fungicides viz., carbendazim or tricyclazole at the rate of 2g/litre of water and soak the seeds in the solution for 2 hrs. Drain the solution and keep the seeds for sprouting

b. Seedling dip / root dip

The seedlings of vegetables and fruits are normally dipped in 0.1% carbendazin or 0.25% copper oxychloride solution for 5 minutes to protect against seedling blight and rots.

c. Rhizome dip

The rhizomes of ginger, cardamom, and turmeric are treated with 0.1% carbendazin solution for 20 minutes to eliminate rot causing pathogen present in the soil.

d. Sett dip / Sucker dip

The sets of sugarcane and tapioca are dipped in 0.1% emisan solution for 30 minutes. The suckers of pine apple may also be treated by this method to protect from soil borne diseases.

(iii) Slurry treatment (Seed pelleting)

In this method, chemical is applied in the form of a thin paste (active material is dissolved in small quantity of water). The required quantity of the fungicide slurry is mixed with the specified quantity of the seed so that during the process of treatment slurry gets deposited on the surface of seeds in the form of a thin paste which later dries up. Almost all the seed processing units have slurry treaters. In these, slurry treaters, the requisite quantity of fungicides slurry is mixed with specified quantity of seed before the seed lot is bagged. The slurry treatment is more efficient than the rotary seed dressers. Eg. Seed pelleting in ragi. Mix 2.5g of carbendazim in 40 ml of water and add 0.5g of gum to the fungicidal solution. Add 2 kg of seeds to this solution and mix thoroughly to ensure a uniform coating of the fungicide over the seed. Dry the seeds under the shade. Treat the seeds 24 hrs prior to sowing.

(iv) Special method of seed treatment

Seed biopriming: Treating of seeds with biocontrol agents and then incubating under warm and moist conditions until just prior to emergence of radical is reffered as bioprimming. This technique has potential advantages over simple coating of seeds as it results in rapid and uniform seedling emergence. *Trichoderma* conidia germinate on the seed surface and form a layer around bioprimed seeds. Such seeds tolerate adverse various soil conditions better. Biopriming could also reduce the amount of biocontrol agents that is applied to the seed.

Procedure of seed biopriming

- Pre soak the seeds in water for 24h.

- Mix the formulated product of *Trichoderma* with the pre-soaked seeds at the rated of 10 g/kg of seed.
- Put the treated seeds as heap.
- Cover the heap with moist jute sac to maintain high humidity.
- Incubate the seeds under high humidity for about 24 h at approximately 25-32^{0}C.
- Bioagents adhered to the seeds grows on the seed surface under moist conditions to form a protective layer all around the seed coat.
- Sow the seeds in nursery beds
- The seeds that bio-primed with bioagents provide protection against seed and soil borne plant pathogens, improving germination and seedling growth.

Model Practice Questions

A. Objective Questions

a. Multiple Choice Questions

1. A compound that temporarily prevents fungus growth or germination without killing the fungus is

(a)	Fugistat	(b)	Fungicide
(c)	Antisporulant	(d)	Antipenetrant

2. Active principle of Bordeaux mixture is

(a)	Copper sulphate	(b)	Calcium sulphate
(c)	Copper hydroxide	(d)	Calcium hydroxide

3. Chestnut compound is prepared with

(a) Copper sulphate and ammonium carbonate

(b) Copper sulphate and ammonium nitrate

(c) Copper sulphate and sodium carbonate

(d) Copper sulphate and sodium nitrate

4. Antifungal antibiotic is

(a)	Griseofulvin	(b)	Blasticidin
(c)	Kasugamycin	(d)	All of these

5.The fungicide isolated from wood rotting mushroom

(a)	Strobilurubins	(b)	Azole
(c)	Morpholine	(d)	Acylalanine

6. The fungicide interfere with mitosis cell division of sensitive fungi is
   (a) Benomyl (b) Carbendazim
   (c) Thiabendazole (d) All the above
7. The group consists of systemic fungicides is
   (a) Bavistin and Captan (b) Plantvax and Emisan
   (c) Bavistin and Calixin (d) Ziram and Blitox
8. Nematicide belongs to carbamate group is
   (a) DBCP (b) DD
   (c) Phorate (d) Aldicarb
9. Fungicide group effective against all the pathogen groups is
   (a) Strobilurins (b) Chlorothalonil
   (c) Dithiocarbamate (d) All of these
10. The fungicide Captan is also called
   (a) Kittelson Killer (b) Giant Killer
   (c) Disease killer (d) Pest killer
11. 'Soda Bordeaux' is
   (a) Bordeaux mixture (b) Chestnut compound
   (c) Burgundy mixture (d) Bordeaux past
12. Khaira disease of rice is controlled by spraying
   (a) Copper sulphate (b) Manganese sulphate
   (c) Borax (d) Zinc sulphate
13. Antisporulent fungicide is
   (a) Bordeaux mixture (b) Captan
   (c) Bavistin (d) Metalaxyl
14. Fungicide showing apoplastic and symplastic movement with in a plant system is
   (a) Fosteyl-Al (b) Captan
   (c) Propiconazole (d) Carboxin
15. Powdery mildew loving fungicide is
   (a) Sulphur (b) Quinolines
   (c) 2-Aminopyrimidines (d) All the above

16. The fungicide grouped under 'High risk category' is
    (a) Benzimidazole (b) Dicarboxamide
    (c) Carbamates (d) Aromatic Hydrocarbon
17. The fungicide interfere with sterol synthesis of sensitive fungi is
    (a) Propiconazole (b) Carbendazim
    (c) Thiabendazole (d) Iprodione
18. The fungicide interfere with DNA and RNA synthesis of sensitive fungi is
    (a) Benomy (b) Carbendazim
    (c) Thiabendazole (d) Iprodione
19. The fungicide interfere with RNA synthesis of sensitive fungi is
    (a) Benomyl (b) Carbendazim
    (c) Thiabendazole (d) Metalaxyl
20. The fungicide inhibit DNA synthesis of sensitive fungi is
    (a) Benomyl (b) Carbendazim
    (c) Thiophanate-methyl (d) All the above

Q. No	Answer	Q. No	Answer
1	(a) Fugistat	11	(c) Burgundy mixture
2	(a). Copper sulphate	12	(d) Zinc sulphate
3	(a) Copper sulphate and ammonium carbonate	13	(a) Bordeaux mixture
4	(d) All of these	14	(a) Fosteyl-Al
5	(a) Strobilurubins	15	(a) Sulphur
6	(d) All the above	16	(a) Benzimidazole
7	(c) Bavistin and Calixin	17	(a) Propiconazole
8	(d) Aldicarb	18	(d) Iprodione
9	(a) Strobilurins	19	(d) Metalaxyl
10	(a) Kittelson Killer	20	(d) All the above

b. True/False

1. Fungicide which is effective only if applied prior to fungal infection is called *protectants*
2. Fungicide which is capable of eradicating a fungus after it has caused infection, and thereby curing the plant, is called *therapeutant* .
3. Usually the chemo-therapeutants are systemic in their action.
4. Contact fungicides are protective in function.
5. Pathogen resistance development commonly not takes place in systemic fungicides.

6. Sulphur fungicides are the oldest chemical of disease control.
7. The most popular fungicides in sulphur groups are the organic compounds known as dithio-carbamates.
8. The fungicide Ediphenphos is very effective against blast of rice.
9. Symplastic movement of fungicides takes place within the non living parts of the cell of plant.
10. Systemic fungicides are either be toxic to the pathogen concerned or be converted in the host plant to such a fungitoxicant.
11. Carboxin was first systemic fungicides to be discovered and introduced for plant disease control.
12. Sterol biosynthesis inhibiting fungicides inhibit *ergosterol biosynthesis* in fungi .
13. Strobilurins are a group of chemical compounds used extracted from the fungus *Strobilurus tenacellus* .
14. Strobilurin are also called QoI inhibitor fungicides.
15. Dusts are free flowing powder contain technical material in the range of 2 to10% inert carrier.
16. Granules are genuine products contain technical material in the range of 3 to 10% and granule base.
17. Aerosols are liquids under pressure filled in cans which on release give a misty spray.
18. Fumigation method is usually used to control plant parasitic nematodes.
19. Seed disinfectants are those which kill the pathogen present on the seed and do not remain active for long after the seed has been planted.
20. Seed disinfestants are those which act as eradicants and destroy the pathogen established in seed tissues.

Answer

Q. No	Answer	Q. No.	Answer
1	True	11	True
2	True	12	True
3	True	13	True
4	True	14	True
5	False	15	True
6	True	16	True
7	True	17	True
8	True	18	True
9	False	19	False
10	True	20	False

6. Descriptive Questions

a. Short answer

1. What is the mode of action of a protectant fungicide?
2. Why protactant fungicides usually provide long term and durable control in comparison to systemic fungicides ?
3. What are the main factors behind pathogen resistance to fungicides?
4. Write down the difference between protactant and systemic fungicides?
5. Why 1960s is considered to be the turning point in the area of chemical treatment of plant diseases?
6. Who discovered Bordeaux mixture? What features make Bordeaux mixture an excellent fungicide?
7. What are the fundamental differences between a systemic fungicide and an antibiotic?
8. Name some important antibiotics used for plant disease management?
9. Who discovered the first dithiobarbamate fungicide? What name was attributed to this fungicide.
10. Mention important features of an ideal systemic fungicide.
11. Name two acylaline fungicides used effectively against Ommycetous fungi?
12. What is antibiotic? Write down advantage and disadvantage of antibiotic in plant disease management.
13. Write down the role of antibiotics in plant disease amangement.
14. Discuss about application technology of chemical in plant disease control.
15. Milestones in the development of fungicides

b. Long answer

1. Write short notes on the following ;
   (a) Sterol biosynthesis inhibitors
   b) Strobilurins
   c) Acylalines
   d) Oxantiins
   e) Organo tin compounds
2. What are systemic fungicides ? Give a detail account of systemic fungicides in plant disease management .

3. What is soil fumigations ? Discuss the role of important soil fumigants in plant disease management.
4. Discuss various application patterns of chemicals in plant disease managment .
5. Gives various methods of classification of fungicides. Support your statement with suitable examples.
6. Enlist important fungicides belonging to organic sulphur group. How mancozeb is toxic to fungi.
7. Write short notes on : a. Characteristic of an ideal fungicide b. Factors affecting the performance of a fungicide.
8. How Bordeaux mixture is prepared ? Describe method, chemical reactions, precaution and advantage of Bordeaux mixture.

19

Integrated Disease Management

The overuse of chemical pesticides and farmers' improper application of them have resulted in a number of issues, including residue in food, feed, and fodder; resistance developing; resurgence, secondary outbreaks; and, most importantly, pollution of the environment. This has caused a condition known as Pesticide Treadmill, which is characterized by the need to apply ever-increasing amounts of chemical pesticides. Integrated Pest/Management was developed as an environmentally sound substitute for the exclusive use of chemicals after Rachel Carson's book "Silent Spring" in 1962 sparked widespread concern about the overuse of pesticides.

The IDM Concept

In disease management, every alternative control strategy—cultural, biological, mechanical, resistant varieties, physical, etc.—is applied in combination to keep the disease below the threshold of economic injury . In order to control the disease, pesticides are employed if it spreads and hits the economic threshold. With consideration for the agro-ecosystem, this approach to integrated disease management uses the minimum amount of pesticides possible. In reality, we don't aim for complete control while managing diseases—rather, we let them progress below what is tolerable, such as the economic threshold. Additionally, it offers agents the chance to endure by controlling the diseases and maintaining a particular state of equilibrium. Therefore, the goal of the integrated disease management concept is to manage the disease using all available strategies while achieving positive effects on the environment, society, and economy.

What is IDM

A farmer-based, intensive management method known as Integrated Disease Management (IDM) promotes disease problems to be naturally managed and stops diseases from escalating to the point where they become economically harmful. Improved natural enemies, disease-resistant crops, cultural management, and, as a last option, the prudent use of pesticides to suppress rather than eradicate the population of target pathogens are all suitable strategies included in the IDM module.

Important Features of IDM

The following are some of the important features of IDM

- IDM is an ecologically sound alternative to chemical disease management. It has also been shown to be economically viable and socially acceptable strategy for disease control for the farmers of our country.
- IDM is consistent with the needs of our agriculture. It provides food security by preventing and reducing crop losses; promotes self reliance by farmer participatory approach thereby, building on their understanding of local agro ecology; contributes to poverty alleviation by focusing on small and marginal farmers and protects environment and health by chemical inputs and conserving bio-diversity.
- The technologies developed have not yet exploited at the level to reach the small and marginal farmers of the country to make IDM as an effective alternative to use of chemical pesticides. Even though successful non chemical methods for the control of crop diseases have been developed, the transfer of this technology to the farmers and extension workers has been rather low. The coverage under IPM a present is estimated to be less than 10 percent of the total cultivable are in the country.
- The wide scale adoption of IDM faces a number of problems. These include the ready availability of appropriate technology and inputs, poor infrastructure and lack of adequate training and education.
- Availability of IDM technology alone is no guarantee that it will prove effective in the field. A top down technology driven approach is unlikely to succeed under Indian conditions .There is therefore, a need for farmers participation, including women, who play a dominant role in both seed selection and crop management

History

Benett(1956) coin the Phrase Integrated control

Geier and clark(1961) used the term Integrated Pest Management

Goals of IDM

The main goal s of an integrated plant disease management programme are to

- Eliminate or reduce the initial inoculums.
- Reduce the effectiveness of initial inoculums.
- Increase the resistance of the host.
- Delay the onset of the disease.
- Slow the secondary cycles.

Objective of IDM

Varied IDM objective are:

- It contributes significantly in the reduction in potential hazards to environment and people health.
- It provides improved control by conservation of natural enemies and employing traditional method.
- It helps in the production of improved quality produce.
- It help to reduce the cost of plant protection and thus render crop protection on economic venture.
- It helps in improvement on water and soil quality.
- It reduces farmers and consumer risk.
- It facilitates better pesticide management.

Framework of IDM strategy

IDM is an holistic guiding principle that encompasses all the activities from selection of crop to the harvest and storage. Broadly speaking, however , IDM strategies are based on thee main pillars.

1. Prevention
2. Monitoring.
3. Intervention.

Most of the IDM activities emphasize heavily on the preventive measures. The first line of defense against disease is prevention through the use of agronomical practices or cultural practices which are unfavorable for the development of disease problems. Regular and sound monitoring of disease is essential for decisions in IDM. Selected control measures to check disease are to be taken at economic threshold level (ETL) or action threshold level (ATL). IDM strives to optimizes rather than maximize pathogen control effects.

Economic injury level: It is the lowest disease index that will cause economic damage.

Economic Threshold level: It is the disease index at which control measures should be applied to prevent an increasing disease from reaching the economic injury level.

Tools of IDM

Monitoring of Diseases: Monitoring is a vital component of an effective IDM program. Monitoring can be direct (looking for the pathogen or disease) or indirect (recording environmental conditions which affect disease development). Financial considerations weigh heavily in the choice of monitoring practice. Direct monitoring of diseases can be based on symptoms or signs of the disease. Identification of pathogens is commonly difficult, because pathogens generally are microscopic and can be detected typically after the disease process has begun. Most monitoring is actually for disease symptoms, with the control strategy aimed at reducing further spread. Even when visible symptoms are evident, levels of disease may be so low as to make detection very tricky. To optimize the chances of detection, one should concentrate on those areas where disease is most likely to occur, for example in low areas or areas of lush growth. If this is not possible, an array of sampling designs may be used, such as a diagonal across the field, a random walk, a stratified design where each subsection of the field is sampled, or a stratified random design where a random sample is taken in each subsection of the field . The appropriate sampling design will depend on the level of disease expected, the distribution of the disease and sampling schemes already in place for other pests. Disease distribution within a field is dependent, in large part, on the source of inoculum for the pathogen. If the disease is seed borne, in many cases the first diseased plants will be more uniformly distributed in the field. If the disease is soil borne, it may often be found in clusters in the field. If it is transmitted by insects, the distribution may be more random, or a field edge effect may be apparent. Thus, it is important to understand the biology of the Indirect monitoring of disease most often involves stand-alone, turn-key computer systems with probes or whole units in the field. Data commonly gathered include temperature, relative humidity, and leaf wetness. Data are typically recorded every fifteen minutes, with data being used to update real time indices of the likelihood of disease at a given time. The algorithms for the models are often developed from controlled environmental chamber experiments where the minimum, maximum, and optimum temperatures and relative humidity for fungal growth, germination, and/or disease development are identified. Leaf wetness, either monitored directly or by prediction of dew point based on the relative humidity and temperature conditions, is used if the pathogen requires free water for germination. The prediction of disease events through environmental monitoring has been very successful in a few cases and is used widely for those crops and diseases where sufficient research exists.

Genetic Host Resistance: The use of genetically resistant plants to minimize or avoid losses caused by insect pests and/or diseases. The use of genetically resistant plants is often recommended by entomologists and plant pathologists as the first line of defense for avoiding or minimizing plant damage caused by insects and pathogens. In some cropping systems, such as large acreage field or row crop agriculture (corn, soybeans wheat, rice, cotton, etc.), the use of genetically resis tant plants may be the only cost-effective means for managing a particular pest or disease. In some cases, the use of resistant cultivars or varieties might be the only means of effectively managing a disease or pest such as in the case of managing plant diseases caused by viruses. The development of resistant plant types may also reduce the need for using pesticides. Although genetic resistance should be considered when dealing annual cropping systems where new seed is sown each season thereby providing an opportunity to introduce new cultivars or varieties with disease resistance. Although important in perennial cropping systems such as orchards, forests, golf courses, or home lawns, once the initial crop is planted, the introduction of resistant lines is limited due to the long-term nature of these crops.

Cultural Control

Cultural practices serve an important role in prevention and management of plant diseases. The benefits of cultural control begin with the establishment of a growing environment that favors the crop over the pathogen. Reducing plant stress through environmental modification promotes good plant health and aids in reducing damage from some plant diseases Sanitation practices aimed at excluding, reducing, or eliminating disease are critical for management of infectious plant diseases. It is important to use only pathogen-free transplants, especially for late blight, bacterial spot, viral diseases and early blight. In order to reduce dispersal of soilborne pathogens between fields, stakes and farm equipment should be decontaminated before moving from one field to the next. Reduction of pathogen survival from one season to another may be achieved by destruction of volunteer plants and crop rotation. Removal of cull piles and prompt destruction of crops should be applied as a general practice. Avoid movement of soil from one site to another to reduce the risk of moving pathogens. For example, sclerotia of *Sclerotinia sclerotiorum* and *Sclerotium rolfsii*, are transported primarily in contaminated soil. Minimizing wounds during harvest and packing will reduce post harvest disease problems. Depending on crops and other factors, sanitation of soil can be achieved to some degree by solarization. Crop rotation is a very important practice, especially for soilborne disease control. For many soilborne diseases, at least a 3-year-rotation using a non-host crop will greatly reduce pathogen populations. This practice is beneficial for Phytophthora blight of pepper and Fusarium wilt of watermelon, but longer rotation periods (up to 5-7 years) may be needed. Land previously cropped to alternate and reservoir hosts should be avoidedwhenever possible. Vegetable fields should be located as far as away as possible from inoculum and insect vector sources. Weed control is important for the management of viral diseases. Weeds may be alternate hosts for several important vegetable viruses and their vectors. Elimination of weeds might reduce primary inoculum. Cover crops help to reduce weed populations that may harbor pathogens between seasons. For this purpose use cover crops that grow fast and provide maximum biomass. Non-host cover crops will help to reduce weed populations and primary inoculum for soilborne pathogens. Excessive handling of plants such as in thinning, pruning and tying may be involved in spread of pathogens, particularly bacteria. It is advisable to handle plants in the field when plants are driest. Because some pathogens can only enter the host through wounds, situations which promote plant injury should be avoided. During pruning process and harvest, workers should periodically clean their hands and tools with a disinfectant, such as isopropyl alcohol. If applicable, plants can be staked and tied for improved air movement in the foliar canopy. A more open canopy results in less wetness discouraging growth of most pathogens. Soil aeration and drying can be enhanced through incorporation of composted organic amendments in the soil. Build up of inoculum can be reduced by removing all plant materials (infected and apparently healthy) after harvest. Between-row cover crops reduce plant injury from blowing sand. Polyethylene mulch can be used as a physical barrier between soil and above-ground parts of plants. This is an important practice for fruit rot control in the field. Highly UV-reflective (metalized) mulches repel some insects. It is beneficial to use metalized mulch during certain times of the year when insect vectors of some viral diseases are prevalent. Tomato spotted wilt virus (TSWV) incidence and associated vector thrips populations have been demonstrated to be effectively reduced by using metalized mulches on tomatoes.

Mechanical control: It involves use of mechanical or manual operation and mechanical barriers for the control of diseases. For example- pruning of diseased part of the plants, rouging of viral infected plants etc. This is especially very effective in high value crops where area under cultivation is less.

Physical control: It involves manipulation of temperature, humidity, lght and sound water etc for controlling diseases. Hot air treatment at 54 °C for 8h, effectively eliminates RSD pathogen without impairing the germination of buds. Similarly, grassy shoot disease of sugarcane has also been controlled by hot air at 54 °C for 8 h.

Biological Control: Biological control is the use of one organism or a group of organisms to suppress, kill, or restrict the activity of a pest or pathogen. The use of biological control is considered advantageous and environmentally sound as it provides an eco-friendly alternative to the use of pesticides. Unfortunately, however, few biocontrol products are available that provide consistent and commercially acceptable levels of pest or disease control.

Biocontrol organisms kill or suppress pathogens and pests by either (a) parasitizing the pathogen, (b) out competing the pest or pathogen for space or nutrients, (c) producing toxins that kill or make pathogen sick, and/or (d) inducing a physiological or biochemical change in the host plant making it less susceptible to (more tolerant of) pathogen attack. Biocontrol agents for use in plant disease management are increasing in use especially among organic growers. These products are considered safer for the environment and the applicator, than conventional chemicals and are mainly used against soilborne diseases. Examples of commercially available biocontrol agents include the fungi *Trichoderma harzianum* and *Gliocladium virens*, an actinomycete *Streptomyces griseoviridis*, and a bacterium *Bacillus subtilis*. Bacteriophages (phages) have been found as an effective biocontrol agent for the management of bacterial spot on tomato. Phages are viruses that infect bacteria. It is best to run small trials on one's own farm to fully evaluate the applicability of biocontrol to particular farming operations.

Regulatory Measures: The use of quarantines and pest eradication programs to limit the introduction or spread of deleterious plant pathogens. Strict government inspections and quarantines of imported plants, plant products, and soil can be an effective way to keep a pathogen out of a region or area. However, given the global nature of modern society, the possibility of moving and introducing diseases dangerous to people, plants, and animals is real. Government eradication programs are conducted when a serious disease breaks out. Often the trouble is eliminated before it has a chance to spread. Such programs require highly trained personnel who know the potential disease problems and are able to recognize the pathogens and the symptoms of their activities. On the grower level, many greenhouses and nurseries also use quarantine measures. They often keep the new material separated from the old. If a disease were to come in on the new material it would not impact the rest of the greenhouse or nursery.

Chemical control: Fungicides and bactericides are an important component of many disease management programs.It is important to remember that chemical use should be integrated with all other appropriate tactics mentioned in this chapter. Information regarding physical mode of action of a fungicide will help producers improve timing of fungicide applications. Physical modes of action of fungicides can be classified into four categories: protective, after infection, pre-symptom, and anti-sporulant (post-symptom). Protectant fungicides include the bulk of the foliar spray materials available to producers. In order to be effective, protectant fungicides, such as copper compounds, mancozeb etc., need to be on the leaf (or plant) surface prior to arrival of the pathogen. Systemic (therapeutic) fungicides, based on their level of systemicity, true systemic (i.e. Aliette), translaminar (i.e. Quadris), meso-systemic (i.e. Flint)], are active inside of the leaf. Systemic fungicides may stop an infection after it starts and prevent further disease development. If necessary fungicides must be used based on recommended fungicide resistance management strategies.A new startegy to chemically manage plant diseases without direct interference with the pathogen is the triggering of plant defense reaction. Acibenzolar-S-methyl (Actigard), a chemical in this category, was registered for the control of bacterial spot and speck on tomatoes. Chemicals must be used at recommended rates and application frequencies. Besides selection of the most efficacious material, equipment must be properly calibrated and attention paid to the appropriate application technique. As always, the key to effective disease management is correct diagnosis of the problem.Always read the pesticide labels and follow the instructions carefully. Remember, the label is the law. Fumigants can be used to manage soilborne pathogens. Before applying, it is important to review the disease history of the specific site when choosing fumigant materials.

Key Components or Steps in the Implementation of IDM:

1. **Correct disease Identification** - What diseases and stages are causing the damage. This is foundation of all decision making.
2. **Understanding of disease and crop dynamics** - Must have enough information about the nature of the pathogens encountered to assess the potential risk that the disease poses and determine the best possible management strategy.
    - How much disease is tolerable?
    - What are the expected losses of the disease if controls are not used?
    - What is the most vulnerable stage for management?
    - Two concepts of importance: window of vulnerability and treatment window
3. **Planning Preventive Strategies** as the preferred management strategy in IDM; a careful examination of field history and all aspects of the crop production system should be made to determine if the crop can be grown or treated to prevent disease from exceeding economic levels.
    - Can any cropping practice, such as time of planting, crop rotation, or tillage, be manipulated to reduce disease attack?
    - Are the chances of economic disease losses great enough to justify a preventive pesticide strategy?
    - What are the benefits and risks of pesticides?

- What are the existing natural control agents that can be augmented or conserved?

4. **Monitoring** - Involves periodic assessment of diseases, natural control factors, crop characteristics, and environmental factors to the need for control and the effectiveness of any management action. Different methods and sampling frequencies are used, depending on the nature of diseases and monitoring objective.
5. **Decision making** - Involves an evaluation of the monitoring information to assess the relevant economic benefits versus the risks of disease management actions. What will I lose if I do nothing? What will I gain?
   - Is there enough natural control agents present to reduce the disease incidence/severity below economic levels?
   - Is the incidence/severity potential of the disease more costly than the control?
   - Estimates of incidence/severity size are compared to "economic thresholds" or "action thresholds" which serve as references for loss potential at particular crop growth stages or sets of crop conditions.
6. **Selection of optimal disease control tactics** to manage the problem while minimizing economic, health and environmental risks.
   - Are there opportunities to integrate nonchemical tactics?
   - How well will the control option fit into the total management system?
   - How well will the tactic control the disease? What effects will this action have on the user, society as a whole, and the environment?
   - Will this action impact, either positively or negatively, the other species or natural enemies present in my crop?

   For chemical controls, important questions at this step are: What is the best fungicide for the target disease? What is the optimal rate? Is it legal? What are the safety requirements and use restrictions?
7. **Implementation** - Once the management options are selected, they should be deployed on a timely manner with precision and completeness. Concept to remember for chemical control: Proper timing and placement is often more important than the rate.
   - What can be done to improve effectiveness of the management tactics?
   - Is the pesticide application equipment calibrated properly and in good working condition?

- If pesticides are used, what is the appropriate chemical and rate for the target disease?
- Can the pesticide be applied in a manner that will be least disruptive on natural enemies while still provide effective control?
- In certain situations, it may be desirable to leave small non-treated areas to evaluate control effectiveness.

8. **Evaluation** - Always take time to follow-up and evaluate disease control actions to determine if you got your money's worth. Review what went wrong but more importantly what went right.
   - Was the choice of control action appropriate?
   - Was the management action implemented on time and according to recommendations?
   - What changes to the management tactics can be made to improve control if the same disease problem occurs in the future?
   - What future changes in the production system can be made to achieve more permanent suppression of the disease problem?

Advantages of IDM

Some of the advantages of an integrated approach are as follows:

- Promotes sound structures and healthy plants.
- Promotes the sustainable bio based disease management alternatives.
- Reduces the environmental risk associated with management by encouraging the adoption of more ecologically benign control tactics.
- Reduces the potential for air and ground water contamination.
- Protects the non-target species through reduced impact of plant disease management activities.
- Reduces the need for pesticides and fungicides by using several management methods.
- Reduces or eliminates issues related to pesticide residue.
- Decreases workers, tenants and public exposure to chemicals.
- Alleviates concern of the public about pest & pesticide related practices.
- Maintains or increases the cost-effectiveness of disease management programs.

Constraints in the Implementation of IDM

A Information and technological constraints

- Through IDM technology in rice, cotton, red gram, certain vegetable etc. is available, there is a lack of multiple resistant varieties.
- There is a need for a number of selective pesticides against diseases of crops which are safe against the natural enemies.
- Economic threshold level information is a crucial requirement for a good IDM package. For the majority of the diseases, these have not been worked out.
- Precise disease surveillance and monitoring methods and forecasting models have not been standardized.
- The techniques of mass multiplication of several potential bio control agents are still not well developed.
- Identifying cropping sequence, plant based pesticides and biocides develop system analysis based plant protection package

B . Institutional constraints

- There is an immense need for multidisciplinary approaches inter institutional collaboration to develop sound IDM technology.
- Human resource development in IDM through training of trainers and farmers.
- Large scale demonstration of field tested IDM policies.
- Participatory approach among state extension functionaries scientists of SAU and research institutes, NGO and farmers group.
- Pesticide industry should also continue their effort to ensure the availability of safe, selective environment friendly and quality pesticides.

Model Practice Questions

A. Objective Questions

a. Multiple Choice Questions

1. Use by of one species of organism to eliminate or control another species of organism ---------------------

(a) IDM	(b) Biological control
(c) Cultural control	(d) Physical control

2. Deep summer ploughing is done mainly for management of diseases ---------------------

(a)	Air borne	(b)	Soil borne
(c)	Seed borne	(d)	None of these

3. An association between species, where one organism lives on or in another organism causing it some harm is called

(a)	Competition.	(b)	Parasitism
(c)	Induction of plant defense	(d)	Antibiosis

4. Soil solarization is an advanced field technology for the management of

(a)	Soil borne pathogens	(b)	Seed borne pathogens
(c)	Air borne pathogens	(d)	All of above

5. Early sowing of chickpea favors the disease

(a)	Collar rot	(b)	Root Rot
(c)	Wilt	(d)	Damping Off

6. A combination of strategies to reduce losses due to disease based on environmental and economic considerations are called

(a)	IDM	(b)	Biological control
(c)	Cultural control	(d)	Physical control

7. The nature of loose smut of wheat is

(a)	Internally seed borne	(b)	Externally seed borne
(c)	Soil born	(d)	All

8. The lowest disease index that can cause economic harm to the crop is called

(a)	Economic injury level	(b)	Economic threshold level
(c)	Pest risk analysis	(d)	None

9. Mixed crops of pigeonpea and sorghum give significant reduction in the incidence of disease of Pigeonpea

(a)	Fusarium wilt	(b)	Root rot
(c)	Collar rot	(d)	Blight

10. The disease index at which control measures should be applied to prevent an increasing disease from reaching the economic injury level

(a)	Economic injury level	(b)	Economic threshold level
(c)	Pest risk analysis	(d)	None

11. Which of the following polythene is most suitable for soil solarization?
    - (a) Black polythene
    - (b) Transparent white polythene
    - (c) Yellow polythene
    - (d) Blue polythene
12. Varieties which escape damage by disease because of their growth characters not due to their genetic resistance to the disease are called
    - (a) Disease escaping varieties
    - (b) Disease excluding varieties
    - (c) Susceptible varieties
    - (d) None
13. The plant which is planted deliberately in the growing area and pest gets attracted to it is called
    - (a) Cash crop
    - (b) Trap crop
    - (c) Sole crop
    - (d) Pitcher crop
14. In India, Destructive Insects and Pests Act, was enacted in
    - (a) 1920.
    - (b) 1914.
    - (c) 1916
    - (d) 1918
15. The national centre for Integrated Pest Management (NCIPM) is located at
    - (a) Hyderabad
    - (b) Chandigarh
    - (c) New Delhi
    - (d) Pune
16. The concept of EIL was proposed by
    - (a) Stern
    - (b) Smith
    - (c) Knipling
    - (d) Bushland
17. Suppressive soils are known to have high population of
    - (a) Antagonistic microorganisms
    - (b) Weeds
    - (c) Propagules of pathogens
    - (d) Nematodes
18. which of the disease management methods is considered as the cheapest, easiest, safest and most effective
    - (a) Biological control
    - (b) Resistant varieties
    - (c) Chemical control
    - (d) Cultural control
19. Bioproduct containing *Ampelomyces quisqualis* AQ10 is effective against which of the following diseases.
    - (a) Powdery mildew
    - (b) Downey mildew
    - (c) Black mildew
    - (d) Late blight

20. An approach to soilborne pest and pathogen management that involves the use of plants primarily from the Brassicaceae family in rotation with cash crops is called

    (a) Biofumigation (b) Greening

    (c) Soil composting (d) Biosuppressing

Answer

Question no	Answer	Question no	Answer
1	(b) Biological control	11	(b) Transparent white polythene
2	(b) Soil borne	12	(a) Disease escaping varieties
3	(b) Parasitism	13	(b) Trap crop
4	(a) Soil borne pathogens	14	(b) 1914.
5	(a) Collar rot	15	(c) New Delhi
6	(a) IDM	16	(a) Stern
7	(a) Internally seed borne	17	(a) Antagonistic microorganisms
8	(a) Economic injury level	18	(b) Resistant varieties
9	(a) Fusarium wilt	19	(a) Powdery mildew
10	(b) Economic threshold level	20	(a) Biofumigation

b. True/False

1. IDM is a sustainable approach to manage diseases by combining biological, cultural, physical and chemical tools in a way that minimizes economic, health and environmental risks.
2. IDM helps to keep a balanced ecosystem.
3. IDM promotes a healthy environment.
4. IDM maintains a good public image.
5. The emphasis in IDM is on management, not eradication.
6. Accurate disease identification is critical to a successful IDM program.
7. Action Threshold Level is a predetermined disease level that is deemed to be unacceptable.
8. There is an immense need for multidisciplinary approaches inter institutional collaboration to develop sound IDM technology.
9. Economic threshold levels have been worked out for the few diseases in India.
10. Suppressive soils are known to have high population of antagonistic microorganisms.
11. The project directorate of biological control (PDPC) is located at Bengaluru.

12. Mixed crops of pigeonpea and sorghum give significant reduction in the wilt disease of Pigeonpea.
13. Use of resistant varieties is considered as the cheapest, easiest, safest and most effective means of disease management.
14. Early sowing of chickpea favors the collar rot disease of chickpea .
15. Black polythene is most suitable for soil solarization.

Question no	Answer	Question no	Answer
1	True	9	True
2	True	10	True
3	True	11	True
4	True	12	True
5	True	13	True
6	True	14	True
7	True	15	False
8	True		

b. Descriptive Questions

Short answer

1. Mention two important problems encountered due to continuous and injudicious use of fungicides?
2. What is IDM?
3. Why IDM is considered to be a system approach?
4. Define EIL, ETL & ATL?
5. Why practice IDM?
6. Wht IDM is considered to be a system approach?

Long Answer

1. What is Integrated Disease Management (IDM), and how does it differ from traditional disease control methods?
2. Explain the role of disease monitoring and early detection in Integrated Disease Management.
3. How do cultural practices contribute to Integrated Disease Management, and what are some examples?
4. What is the role of biological control agents in Integrated Disease Management, and how are they used?
5. Discuss the challenges associated with integrating chemical control into an Integrated Disease Management plan.

6. How does Integrated Disease Management address environmental sustainability?
7. What are the economic benefits of adopting Integrated Disease Management in agricultural systems?
8. How can Integrated Disease Management strategies be adapted for different regions or agricultural systems?
9. What are the key principles and steps involved in developing an Integrated Disease Management plan?
10. Explain the role of education and farmer involvement in the successful implementation of Integrated Disease Management.